Praise for *Health Care Revolt*

"*Health Care Revolt* by Dr. Michael Fine is a critical read about what we need to do for the future of our health care system in America. In Central Falls we have now experienced the benefits of a Neighborhood Health Station that has the capacity to serve the majority of the community and focus on preventive care. This model focuses on tackling health care issues from a grassroots level."
  —James A. Diossa, mayor of Central Falls, Rhode Island

"Michael Fine is one of the true heroes of primary care over several decades."
  —Dr. Doug Henley, CEO and executive vice president of the American Academy of Family Physicians

"Dr. Fine's prose carries a clarity and sense of urgency that are motivating to an increasingly impatient profession and public. This book should inspire the nation to make a break with the same old political mess that is bankrupting Americans and undermining our democracy."
  —David H. Bor, MD, chief academic officer, Cambridge Health Alliance

"Michael Fine has given us an extraordinary biopic on health care in America based on the authority of his forty-year career as writer, community organizer, family physician, and public health official. In *Health Care Revolt*, he channels the core frustration felt by so many, providing a compelling commentary for a nation confused about which health care direction to travel."
  —Fitzhugh Mullan, professor of health policy in the Milken Institute School of Public Health at George Washington University

"Michael Fine is angry. His frustration with the U.S. health care system runs deep and so does his prescription for reform. That prescription means understanding how poorly we are served by our non-system. It means understanding how money drives our non-system. And it means understanding how its reform depends on all of us working together locally and nationally, motivated by a new vision of health. All that and more is in this passionate, fierce book."

—Christopher F. Koller, president, Milbank Memorial Fund

"As Rhode Island's Director of Health, Dr. Fine brought a vision of a humane, local, integrated health care system that focused as much on health as on disease and treatment. Dr. Fine is proposing a new, smart approach to how we think about health care and the connection between burdensome medical costs and the well-being of our democracy."

—U.S. Senator Sheldon Whitehouse

"In the early 1700s, twelve people came together to meet over a printing shop in London. The twelve shared a passion to eliminate the slave trade in the British Empire at a time when all wealth in the Empire derived from slave trade–related businesses. It took them forty years to accomplish their goal. Dr. Fine has laid out and substantiated the argument that the U.S. lacks a health care system. He also describes what a health care system might look like. Further he argues that those of us in the know—and especially the physicians—need to lead the effort to create something better for our current generation and for generations to come. So who else is in? Let's do this thing."

—Laurence Bauer MSW, MED, Family Medicine Education Consortium

HEALTH CARE REVOLT

How to Organize,
Build a Health Care System,
and Resuscitate Democracy—
All at the Same Time

Michael Fine

Foreword by Bernard Lown
and Ariel Lown Lewiton

362.1
FIN
col

PMPRESS

Health Care Revolt: How to Organize, Build a Health Care System, and Resuscitate Democracy—All at the Same Time
Michael Fine

© Michael Fine 2018
This edition © PM Press 2018

PM Press
PO Box 23912
Oakland, CA 94623
www.pmpress.org

ISBN: 978-1-62963-581-1
Library of Congress Control Number: 2018931522

10 9 8 7 6 5 4 3 2 1

Printed in the USA

Contents

Acknowledgments

THIS BOOK IS BASED ON MANY YEARS OF MEDICAL PRACTICE, HEALTH CARE POLICY development, and health care administration. Many people helped me, including numerous colleagues: the faculty and residents of Brown University / Memorial Hospital Residency Program in Family Medicine; colleagues at Hancock County Tennessee Health Department; at Hillside Avenue Family and Community Medicine; at the Scituate Health Alliance; at the Rhode Island Adult Correctional Institution Medical Department; at the Rhode Island Department of Health; in the City of Central Falls; and at Blackstone Valley Health Care, Inc. Many people taught me: Tom Gilbert, MD, Steve Davis, MD, Ester Entin, MD, Larry Culpepper, MD, Jack Cunningham, MD, Vince Hunt, MD, and many others. I've had the opportunity to know and work with many great physicians and nurses: Lynn Blanchette, RN and PhD, Elizabeth Gilbertson, RN, Frank Basile, MD, James McDonald, MD, Arnold Goldberg, MD, Solmaz Betash, MD, Pam Harrop, MD, Josh Gutman, MD, Colin Harrington, MD, Jody Rich, MD, Jeffery Brenner, MD, Jim Tomarkin, MD, Don Weaver, MD, Fitzhugh Mullan, MD, Maclaren Baird, MD, Neil Calman, MD, Paul Grundy, MD, Kurt Stange, MD and PhD, and countless others. I've had amazing heroes and mentors: Jack Medalie, MD, Barbara Starfield, MD, H. Jack Geiger, MD, David Satcher, MD and PhD, and Bernard Lown, MD, the coauthor of the Foreword and a major influence on my life and thinking.

In 1999, I was lucky enough to receive a fellowship from the Open Society Institute Program on Medicine as a Profession, now known as the Institute on Medicine as a Profession. David Rothman, PhD, has led that organization for many years and has done more to create light in what is sometimes an anti-intellectual profession than anyone I know. My association with the other IMAP fellows these past twenty years has been satisfying, enlightening, and sustaining, and has helped me to think critically about health, health care, and society. In 2009, I was lucky enough to spend a month as a senior scholar at the Robert Graham Institute in Washington and work with Robert Phillips, MD, Andrew Bazemore, MD, and Stephen Petterson, PhD, who taught me how to think and write about health policy in a new way. In 2011, I was lucky enough to become a member of ASTHO, the Association of State and Territorial Health Officers, and to join with a group of committed public health professionals from across the political spectrum. My ASTHO colleagues taught me to challenge many assumptions, as together we focused on improving the nation's health. In 2015, I was lucky enough to join the board of the Lown Institute.. My board colleagues have been a source of inspiration, calm, and wisdom in troubling times. Governor Lincoln Chafee let me run the Rhode Island Department of Health and was always willing to listen and respond to public health emergencies. Stephanie Chafee lent incredible support for public health during my years in government. George Nee and Ira Magaziner were always present in the background, ready to help.

Sam Mirmirani, PhD, helped me write my first policy paper and was always there to bounce around ideas. James Peters coauthored my first book and helped me think more clearly about ideas and writing. Larry Bauer, MSW, Sandy Blount, EdD, and Doug Henley, MD, encouraged, fomented, and inspired me. Jeff Borkan, MD, and I have been quiet allies for a very long time. Chris Koller has been a partner and teacher for more than twenty-five years. He taught me how to think about primary care policy and how government works, but even more than that, he taught me the quiet wisdom of incremental change, a quiet wisdom this book disregards at its own peril. Shannon Brownlee, quiet revolutionary that she is, taught me the value of unrelenting intellectual courage and the importance of camaraderie and solidarity in the face of what still promises to be a very long struggle. Paul Stekler has listened to me for longer than I can imagine, listened to me rant about health policy and social justice for forty years and still somehow sounds interested in these ideas whenever I talk about them. Lindsey Lane encouraged me to write this book. Jim Tull and Camilo Viveiros helped me remember community organizing and to revive the organizer that lay dormant inside me for many years.

Jennifer Pool Miller talked openly and honestly with me about her daughter Caroline's harrowing bout with the flu. Serese Marotta of Families Fighting Flu was invaluable in facilitating that conversation. Frank Lalli helped me think through finding a publisher.

The work of Wendell Berry has had a major influence on this book. His thinking about the interdependence of community and how meaning comes from community shaped many of these ideas.

Carol Levitt, MD, has stood beside me for every moment of the last thirty-nine years. I would not have been able to write this book, or even to have lived this life, without her. Gabriel and Rosie Fine grew up listening to all this. They can make these arguments better than I can, and their support and love has kept me (almost) sane. Rosie helped me tremendously with this manuscript, proofreading and critiquing the first draft.

But I still learn the most from the people I've had the honor of caring for as patients. I tried to listen. I hope they got back from me some small fraction of the huge amount I learned from them.

Foreword
Bernard Lown, MD, and Ariel Lown Lewiton

THE UNITED STATES IS A NATION DEEPLY DIVIDED, A PREEXISTING CONDITION that has been radically exacerbated in the Trump era. There may be only one point on which almost all Americans agree: that our health care system is profoundly broken. Daily the media report horror stories relating to our dysfunctional health care.

This breakdown is commonly attributed to runaway costs, a persuasive narrative repeated by government, the media, and members of our own profession. In 1957, annual health spending was approximately $147 per person. It has now reached $11,000 per person per year—$3.2 trillion overall—more than double the cost of health care in any other industrialized nation. We currently spend about 30 percent of our average household income on health insurance and medical care. The Congressional Budget Office estimates that if health costs continue to rise at their present rate, by 2025 they'll consume 50 percent of the average family's income, and *100 percent* by 2035.

This is clearly an unsupportable scenario. Americans generally understand that medical care has become a huge industry, a hospital-centered sickness system, driven principally by financial incentives, with little concern for the actual health of the populace. Yet inexorable cost escalation is only one of the many afflictions ailing health care in the United States. The striking shift from primary to specialist care has exacted multiple adverse consequences including an escalation of procedures,

excessive and unnecessary prescribing, and a near-erotic infatu-
ation with technology. These encourage overtreatment, undertreatment, and mistreatment.

The current system of medical education, with its obsessive
focus on science and technology, leaches the profession of its
compassion and idealism. Upon entering medical school, most
first-year students are eager to do good for others. Once students
reach their third year, where training largely takes place in hospitals burgeoning with sophisticated and costly technologies, their
career goals begin to shift toward doing well for themselves.
No wonder a majority of matriculating young doctors choose
to concentrate on lucrative specialties rather than prevention-
focused primary care.

Another major flaw in our health care infrastructure is the
scarcity of funding devoted to preventative services. It should be
obvious that the most effective way to save on health care costs
is to focus on preventing people from getting sick in the first
place. Preventative care is not just a matter of public health: it
includes safe and affordable housing, sanitation, access to clean
water and nutritious food, reliable public transportation, and
education. Yet those who argue most vehemently for health care
reform on the grounds of escalating costs are largely silent about
the centrality of public health. This stance is both economically
perverse and devoid of medical rationale.

After the emergence of the British National Health Service in
1948, many other industrialized democracies adopted some sort
of single-payer arrangement. The fundamental principle of this
system is that health care is a right, not a privilege. Meanwhile,
Americans tend to subscribe to the philosophy that we pay more
in order to get more. The United States has the most expensive health care in the world, yet Americans are far from the
healthiest—we lag unconscionably far behind other countries in
important health indicators such as life expectancy and infant
and maternal mortality rates.

Health care in the United States is exorbitantly costly, exploitative, and inadequate. Most Americans know this yet have tolerated it for a number of reasons, including the massive medicalization of thinking, a childish faith in the magic of technology, and a deeply ingrained sense of futility, in no small measure due to deep distrust of the goings-on in Washington. At the same time, numerous polls show that the majority of Americans support some sort of a single-payer system. Most Americans, physicians and patients alike, believe that health care is a right, not a privilege.

We can and must leverage this ideological support into concrete action. We need to emphasize the centrality of the patient in all our deliberations, all our actions, and all our solutions. Providing people with the medical care they deserve is a moral imperative. We in the health profession must be agents of deep systemic change. Rather than attempting to beseech politicians or sway the various vested interests that control health care, our objective must reach across economic, ethnic, cultural, and social divides in order to mobilize a wide public to compel action.

At the same time, even if we were able to enact a national health plan, we would not have solved what ails American health care. We would still have to restore the patient's rightful place at the center of healing. We would still have to switch away from hospitals as the mainstays of sickness care. We would still have to incorporate effective human communication into medical school curricula and emphasize the role of psychosocial stress as dominant risk factors in all that ails humans. We would still have to invest heavily in preventive medicine and in palliative care. We would still have to quench the culture of overtreatment.

And we would have to continue to confront inequality as the leading cause of disease domestically and globally. Inequality is a fundamental issue of our time, encompassing economic inequality, racial inequality, gender inequality, and health inequality. Doctors are aware that the sickest among us are those who live in poverty. In 2016, more than forty million Americans lived below the poverty line, and one-third of those were children. The World Health Organization has long emphasized that poverty is the leading cause of disease. Undertreatment is a dominant moral issue of our time.

To implement structural changes on this scale is no easy feat, and in *Health Care Revolt* Dr. Michael Fine has provided us with an invaluable primer and guide to action. With the sharp precision of the scientist and the accumulated wisdom of the experienced clinician, Dr. Fine delivers a university education in nine concise and informative chapters. *Health Care Revolt* details how health care in the United States went astray to become a "wealth extraction system" dominated by market forces, with a primary objective of lining the pockets of executives, shareholders, and corporations, rather than improving the health of its citizens.

Dr. Fine goes beyond diagnosis to craft an intimate and comprehensive guide for how we might go about fixing our broken health care system. In doing so, he invokes an element far too often omitted from discussions of health care: the vitality and centrality of public health.

Exploring the history and development of diverse health care models in the twentieth and early twenty-first century, Dr. Fine takes us to Mound Bayou, Mississippi, where Dr. Jack Geiger and social worker John Hatch built a rural community health center in 1967 that sought to address the most urgent needs of the population through integrated medical and public health services. The Tufts-Delta Health Center became a model for community health centers, which now provide medical care to twenty-five million Americans.

Dr. Fine then transports us across the globe to North Karelia, Finland, which had the highest rate of heart disease death in the world until 1972, when the Ministry of Health sent a public health physician, Pekka Puska, and his team to address the problem at its root. Through a multitude of public health initiatives—including exercise and wellness programs, smoking cessation programs, and changes in diet and food production—the community members were able to transform their lifestyles and health, and today Finland boasts some of the best health outcomes in the world.

And we travel to Dr. Fine's home of Central Falls, Rhode Island, where he and other community leaders have built a Neighborhood Health Station that provides fully integrated services for community members, ranging from transportation to housing to drug counseling to urgent care, and offers a blueprint for how other communities across the United States can take their health into their own hands.

Above all, Michael Fine reminds us that health care and democracy are inextricably linked. "Democracy requires that our people be healthy enough to speak for themselves," he writes. "A political revolution in health care is both democracy in action and exactly how we can bring democracy back to life."

For every revolution, we seek a prophetic voice to clarify our struggle and articulate our way forward. In 1775, Thomas Paine's pamphlet *Common Sense* served as the rallying cry for the colonists who craved representative, egalitarian governance and were willing to go to battle for it. Today, with a trumpet in hand, Michael Fine is sounding the call once again. May *Health Care Revolt* serve as the *Common Sense* of our present moment.

From the long view of history, there would be little progress if people did not demand and struggle for the seemingly unobtainable. The people are arbiters of history. This is reflected in the long democratic story of our country. It is affirmed the world over. The agents of change are many, but it is incumbent upon medical professionals to lead the charge for revolutionary change in health care, which we begin by insisting that medicine is a calling, not a business. Rudolf Virchow, one of the giants of nineteenth-century health care, wrote: "Medicine is a social science and politics is nothing more than medicine on a grand scale." He believed that physicians were the natural attorneys for the sick, as well as the poor and the afflicted. By joining forces with patients and communities, we can achieve the ambitious goals that Michael Fine lays out in this text. We are not unmindful that human beings are complex amalgams of mind, emotion, spirituality, and a deeply imbedded morality. We need to excite the entire neural network. We can and must become the catalysts of change—for our health and for our democracy.

BERNARD LOWN IS PROFESSOR EMERITUS OF CARDIOLOGY AT the Harvard School of Public Health and the developer of the direct current defibrillator. As a peace activist he cofounded the International Physicians for the Prevention of Nuclear War, an organization that won the Nobel Peace Prize in 1985. He is the author of *The Lost Art of Healing: Practicing Compassion in Medicine* and *Prescription for Survival: A Doctor's Journey to End Nuclear Madness.*

ARIEL LOWN LEWITON IS A WRITER AND EDITOR BASED IN New York. Her essays, stories, and criticism have appeared in the *Los Angeles Review of Books*, the *National, Vice*, the *Paris Review Daily, Tin House* online, and elsewhere. She has an MFA from the University of Iowa's Nonfiction Writing Program and is a contributing editor at *Guernica* magazine.

We Are Missing the Point:
We've Got a Market, Not a Health Care System

THE VIRUS WE NOW KNOW AS HIV WAS FIRST ISOLATED IN 1983. HIGHLY ACTIVE antiretroviral therapy, very much like the treatment we use today, was discovered in 1996. This made HIV a treatable disease that relatively few people now die from. Once we know that a person has the virus, we get that person on medicine and help them stay on it, which keeps the virus from making the person sick and also blocks the spread of HIV to anyone else. Treatment of HIV-infected people turns out to be a particularly effective way to prevent HIV transmission. In fact, if HIV treatment were a vaccine, it would be the most effective vaccine we have. In theory, all we have to do to end the HIV epidemic in the U.S. is to find every person with HIV in the nation, get each person on treatment, and maintain them in treatment. If we do that, the transmission of HIV inside the United States stops. Forever. No more new cases, other than those imported from other countries. No fears about accidental transmission from toilet seats or blood transfusions or kissing. No more horrible deaths. It turns out that we don't actually need a vaccine to stop the spread of HIV. We can end the HIV epidemic tomorrow using the science we have today.

"What a miracle!" you might say. "We recognized a complex and deadly new disease and discovered the tools we needed to eliminate it in just fifteen years. HIV is history, right?" But if you think that, you're sadly mistaken. Even though we have the tools we need to eliminate HIV, we are not even close to eradicating it. The Centers for Disease Control estimates that between 35,000 and 50,000 Americans are newly infected with HIV each year, but only 20,000 of those are diagnosed. And there are currently over 150,000 Americans who have the virus, are able to transmit it, but don't yet know they are infected.[1]

We have a way to treat HIV and prevent its spread! And we've had those tools since 1996! How is it that HIV still exists?

HIV still exists because, though we have all the *scientific* tools we need to eradicate it, we don't have the organization we need to activate all that science: we don't have a health care system. We have water. We just don't have the pump.

In order to eliminate HIV in the U.S., we need to test the blood of all Americans. We have a social security and tax system that can identify every American who needs to pay taxes and a selective service system that identifies and classifies every American of age for military service, but we don't have a way to find every American who hasn't been tested for HIV.

Even if we had a way to identify and find every American who needs testing, we still have no way to get to those Americans who haven't been tested yet. The Centers for Disease Control and Prevention (CDC) recommends testing every American adult for HIV, but there is no organization or agency to make that happen or even to track our progress. We have an education system that ensures every American child will be given a basic elementary and high school education, but we don't have a system to arrange to draw blood or take a little sample of saliva from all the people who need HIV testing. We have no way to record which people have been tested already and no system that keeps going

---

1   Centers for Disease Control and Prevention, "HIV / AIDS: Basic Statistics," December 18, 2017, available at https://www.cdc.gov/hiv/basics/statistics.html (accessed April 29, 2018).

until every American adult is tested. What's more, we have no system to make sure that everyone who tests positive for HIV gets into treatment and no system to make sure that everyone being treated for HIV stays in treatment. So there are 150,000 Americans walking around with HIV who don't know it and are infecting others every time they have sex or share needles.

The process of reducing the burden of HIV in the U.S. has become the process of designing work-arounds to deal with the health care system we don't have. Instead of identifying every HIV-positive American, getting them on treatment, and maintaining them on treatment, public health and other health professionals find ways of doing what we euphemistically call "harm reduction." That's public health speak for doing the best we can in a nation without a health care system. We create needle exchange programs to give fresh needles to people who shoot drugs so they don't transmit the virus to one another by sharing works. We send health care workers into bathhouses and put advertisements on the apps people use to find anonymous sexual partners, urging people to practice safe sex and to get tested. Sometimes we try to talk people out of having sex with multiple partners, and some of us think we might be able to talk people who are not married out of having sex at all—a work-around that makes theoretical but not practical sense in a culture that endlessly markets sex and uses sex to sell almost everything. We've created a special set of social services and federally funded health services for people with HIV once it has been diagnosed—services that are critically important to people living with HIV—but these programs are something of a distraction from the perspective of prevention policy. These programs allow politicians and the public to think that we are preventing most HIV transmission, when the only truly effective prevention is the prevention we would accomplish if we were to test all Americans adults, find everyone who is infected, get them on treatment, and maintain them in treatment. Build a health care system, and we wouldn't need work-arounds, because we'd eliminate native transmission of HIV in the United States.

We don't actually need to do that much more research into HIV. We have all the science we need to stop the epidemic tomorrow, but we don't have a health care system that can coordinate the work required.

That's because we don't have a health care system at all.

What is a health care system anyway? We have lots of people who make a living from health care—doctors and nurses, hospitals and clinics, health insurance companies and government bureaucrats, pharmaceutical companies and pharmaceutical retailers, and medical device manufacturers and home health agencies that are running around in communities dispensing health care services and products. Isn't that a health care system?

No. People selling services and products isn't a system. It's a market.

A health care system is an organized set of services and products made available to the entire population and designed to achieve a predetermined set of outcomes. We have water supply systems in most American communities that deliver relatively safe and relatively pure water to every household. We have a public safety system that delivers fire and police protection and functions according to certain standards for everyone in the communities they serve. We have a public education system that makes elementary and high school education available without charge to every child in all American communities. But we have no health care system. No one decides what health care services every American should have. No one sets standards for those universally available services. No one figures out how we are going to make sure every American gets those services, and no one figures out how we are going to pay for what we believe every American should have. In fact, what passes for health care reform in the U.S. is a seemingly endless debate about how we are going to pay for the products and services that are available in the market. We never discuss what products and services we all need and how they are to be supplied equally to everybody. And we experience different versions of the problem that we have with HIV for lots of diseases and conditions. We know how to prevent most heart disease and stroke. We know how to eliminate colon cancer and cervical cancer. To end unplanned adolescent pregnancy. To reduce infant mortality by more than half. We don't apply much of what we know, because we don't have a systemic approach to bringing those scientifically proven prevention services to all Americans.

We don't know who all our smokers are, so we can't reach out to every smoker to help them quit. We don't know everyone struggling with substance use, so we can't bring treatment and recovery services to all of those five to six million Americans. We don't have a list of everyone with high cholesterol. Or diabetes. Or high blood pressure. Many people haven't even been tested for high cholesterol or diabetes or high blood pressure, because we have no way to know who has been tested and who hasn't. In fact, the huge number of people who have undiagnosed high cholesterol, diabetes, and high blood pressure is a major public health threat, a situation people at the CDC worry about all the time. Even if we could identify everyone who needs prevention, we have no way to make that prevention happen. No way to test everyone untested for high blood pressure, diabetes, and high cholesterol. And no way to treat the people we identify.

We have a market, not a system, a market that is not particularly effective at improving the population's health but is egregiously expensive. In 2003, about 17 percent of household income was spent on health insurance and medical services. In 2017, we spent about 30 percent of household income on health insurance and medical services, so that we now spend as much for medical care as we do for housing. The best estimate is that we waste about 30 percent of what we spend on unnecessary or dangerous medical services, although comparisons to other countries suggest we waste 50 to 70 percent of what we spend, with the end result that between $1 trillion and $2 trillion dollars a year is being skimmed off the top as profit. At $11,000 per person per year, which is about the average cost of health care in the U.S., we are wasting $3,000 per person per year or more—$12,000 for a family of four, almost the cost of a new car every year or the cost of a very fancy vacation. The cost of a college education for two kids, if that putative family of four banked the 12K a year for eighteen years.

It's estimated that by 2025 we'll be spending 50 percent of household income on health insurance and medical services. By 2032, we will spend an estimated 100 percent of the average family income on health care.[2] I hope you understand how that will work, because I don't. Neither does any economist. Think climate change is a threat to our planet? It is, but many believe that climate change will take fifty to a hundred years to destroy the planet. Health care is on track to destroy our economy and our nation within fifteen years.

At the same time this medical services market is also draining resources needed for other essential public services. Health care cost inflation has been running 4 to 12 percent for the last thirty years—two to three times the general level of inflation.[3] At $3.2 trillion—our yearly health care spending—we spend an extra $192 billion *every year* just to maintain the health services

2   Richard A. Young and Jennifer E. DeVoe, "Who Will Have Health Insurance in the Future?" *Annals of Family Medicine* 10, no. 2 (March–April 2012): 156–62.

3   Aaron C. Catlin and Cathy A. Cowan, "History of Health Spending in the United States, 1960–2013," November 19, 2015, available at https://www.cms.gov/Research-Statistics-Data-and-Systems/Statistics-Trends-and-Reports/NationalHealthExpendData/Downloads/HistoricalNHEPaper.pdf (accessed April 28, 2018).

we currently supply for the people who currently have access to those services. That is about one-quarter of everything the U.S. spends on public education in a year. Total spending on public housing in 2015 was $190 billion.[4] Imagine what our education system would look like if we could spend an extra $192 billion per year on education? Imagine what would happen to homelessness if we doubled our spending on public housing?

The market is doing exactly what we ask a market to do—maximizing profit. Our health care corporations—insurers, pharmaceutical companies, hospital holding companies, and the like—make billions of dollars in profits and some doctors and health care executives are making salaries in the millions of dollars, but most Americans haven't had a raise in years. Money that should come out of the economy as wage growth that could improve the lives of working people instead produces profit for health care corporations and their shareholders.

And all that money doesn't buy us much health. The United States spends twice as much on medical services as the average spent by other industrialized countries but gives us a population health that ranks us forty-third to fifty-fifth in the world.[5] Our health scientists and biotechnology companies lead the world in product development, but our public health outcomes aren't very good. Our infant mortality rate is three times the best achievable rate in the world. Our life expectancy is five years less than nations with the most effective health care systems. We are paying two to four times what the nations with the best health

4   Center for Budget and Policy Priorities, "Chart Book: Federal Housing Spending Is Poorly Matched to Need," March 8, 2017, available at http://www.cbpp.org/research/housing/chart-book-federal-housing-spending-is-poorly-matched-to-need (accessed April 12, 2018).

5   Central Intelligence Agency, "Country Comparison: Life Expectancy at Birth," The World Factbook, available at https://www.cia.gov/library/publications/the-world-factbook/rankorder/2102rank.html (accessed April 29, 2018).

outcomes pay per person per year, yet we have huge disparities in health outcomes by race, location, and incomes. Health
outcomes for African American men who live in inner cities are
worse than the health outcomes of the world's poorest nations.
The infant mortality rate for African American infants is three to
four times higher than the infant mortality rate for white infants,
which is itself three times higher than the best infant mortality
rates in the world.

Having a market instead of a health care system also un-
dermines democracy. Our democracy depends on our ability
to provide a level of function for all Americans. In order for
democracy to work, citizens have to be healthy enough to speak,
to vote, to write letters to the editor or op-eds, to run for town
council, to testify at the state legislature, and to run for Congress
or president. Democracy requires that our people be healthy
enough to speak for themselves. But because we don't have a
health care system, too many people—limited by illness, injury,
or poverty—are unable to speak up or even act up. Even worse,
because we have a market and not a health care system, some of
the money extracted gets used by people with something to sell,
as they lobby Congress or buy influence in the political process,
which increasingly favors the voices of the few. A health care
system that is for people, not for profit, protects democracy by
enabling more people to participate in the democratic process,
and it protects democracy by cutting off some of the excess profit
that gets used to tilt the playing field toward those who are making plenty of money already.

The purpose of this book is to help Americans understand what
a health care system is, what a health care system would look
like, how a health care system works, and why having a health
care system would be an effective and affordable way to provide
health care to all Americans. Along the way, I'll argue that our
current approach, which uses the market as a way to distribute

medical services, is making us sicker and poorer, and I'll show you how using the market, instead of a health care system is endangering the public's health, disrupting our economy, and undermining our democracy. I'll tell you about a few—out of thousands—of instances where the market allowed health care profiteers to legally steal billions of dollars from the public. I'll tell you about some brave health care pioneers who have tried to build health care systems in some of our neighborhoods and communities and how the market, our jurisprudence, and our politics wrecked those experiments. And I'll tell you what successful, healthy countries do—countries that have great public health outcomes and pay about a quarter of what we pay for health care, using their health care systems to create a healthy population without breaking the bank.

I'll talk a lot about cost and about democracy. While it isn't possible to prove that money wasted on health care is itself contributing to the erosion of our public life, it is also hard to ignore what is happening to our democracy. I'll argue that health and democracy are inextricably linked, noting that the great advances in public health, doubling life expectancy and decreasing infant mortality 250-fold, have occurred in progressive democracies, and that those democracies drive public health improvements around the world. I'll reflect on how health is an essential service in a democracy, because the health of the citizenry is necessary for the public process of democracy to work. And I'll detail the risks to democracy that the health care market creates as it allows wealth to be concentrated in a few hands, where it can be used to tilt decision-making and direct public spending away from the public good.

I'll talk about Obamacare and Trumpcare and about how to create a political revolution in health care that can and will build a health care system to serve all Americans. Think Obamacare fixed it? Think again. Obamacare didn't scratch the surface of what we need to do together if we are going to fix this mess.

And if it was a mess before Congress started its DIY approach to health care reform, it's going to be ten times messier before it's done.

We can do better than Obamacare—much better. The real purpose of this book is to help you understand what "better" looks like—what a health care system is, who it serves, why it matters, and how we can stand up together and get that health care system built. The real purpose of this book is to get health care workers and members of the public to stand up together and revolt and build a health care system from the ground up.

And reinvigorate our precious democracy in the process.

Before we lose it.

CHAPTER ONE

What Are We Doing Wrong?

WE SPEND $3.2 TRILLION PER YEAR ON HEALTH CARE, TWICE AS MUCH AS THE average industrialized country, and three to four times as much as countries with the best public health in the world.[1] But our public health outcomes that rank us no better than forty-third in the world. That's like picking up two dollars worth of eggs, getting charged four dollars at the checkout counter, and then getting home to find out half your eggs are broken. For $3.2 trillion a year, we should have the longest life expectancy in the world, but we are ranked thirteenth among the thirteen industrialized democracies and forty-third in the world. For $3.2 trillion a year, we should have the lowest infant mortality in the world, but we are ranked thirteenth among the thirteen industrialized democracies and thirty-seventh in the world. And for $3.2 trillion a year, we should have no measurable health disparities among population groups who differ only by skin color, language, or geography. In the little state of Rhode Island, which is only forty miles long and twenty miles wide, some population groups have infant mortality rates that are twice as high as others.[2] Some

---

1 David Squires and Chloe Anderson, "U.S. Health Care from a Global Perspective," *The Commonwealth Fund*, available at http://www.commonwealthfund.org/publications/issue-briefs/2015/oct/us-health-care-from-a-global-perspective (accessed April 28, 2018).

2 *Rhode Island Kids Count Factbook*, 2018, 72–73 available at http://www.rikidscount.org/Portals/0/Uploads/Documents/Factbook%202018/2018%20Factbook.pdf (accessed April 29, 2018).

places have rates of adolescent pregnancy that are ten times higher than others.[3] Some people with darker skin tones have life expectancies that are five years shorter than others.[4] As with everyone else in the country, we spend about $11,000 per person per year to achieve these dismal outcomes.[5]

Most experts think about a third of what we spend on health care—a trillion dollars a year—is unnecessary, dangerous, fraudulently obtained, or wasteful. If you compare us to other industrialized countries with similar standards of living, many experts think that number is much larger, that we might actually be wasting half of our spending, or $1.5 trillion a year.

Why do we waste that much?

First, we spend money on the wrong stuff.

We spend money on hospitals and drugs and doctors at a rate that is twice the rate of inflation, but doctors and drugs and hospitals don't have much influence on health. Doctors and drugs and hospitals might keep you from dying today or tomorrow when you get sick, but that doesn't change how long you will live by more than a few days or weeks or how healthy your baby will be. Other people and other factors influence health much more than medicine. Education, housing, public transportation, the time people spend together, and the extent to which we trust each other are all constructs that are associated with a healthier population.

Beyond that, we've allowed ourselves to focus on profits from the health care enterprise instead of understanding the

---

3   *Rhode Island Kids Count Factbook*, 2018, 84–85.

4   U.S. data, not specifically measured for Rhode Island; "State Health Facts: Life Expectancy at Birth (in Years) by Race / Ethnicity," *KFF*, available at https://www.kff.org/other/state-indicator/life-expectancy-by-re/?current Timeframe=0&sortModel=%7B%22colId%22:%22Location%22,%22sor t%22:%22asc%22%7D (accessed April 29, 2018).

5   "National Per Capita Health Expenditure in the United States from 1960 to 2018 (in U.S. Dollars)," Statista, available at https://www.statista. com/statistics/184955/us-national-health-expenditures-per-capita-since-1960/ (accessed April 28, 2018).

way our culture creates dysfunction and disease. We promote products that sicken and kill people instead of promoting a healthy population that strengthens communities and supports democracy.

Consider diabetes. Diabetes is a major driver of health care costs and causes lots of heart disease, kidney failure, and blindness. The good news is that we have plenty of good drugs to treat diabetes, some of which are even still affordable despite the disgusting attempts by venture capital companies to use patent law, market power, and the regulatory process to make drugs that are cheap to produce unimaginably expensive. The better news is that most diabetes is preventable and can be controlled by diet and weight loss, because most diabetes occurs in people who are overweight. But what we do now, of course, is publicly subsidize farmers who grow the corn and wheat from which we manufacture overly processed, high-calorie food-like goop, and then we market the hell out of these high-calorie foods to over-tired Americans, so people eat too much of the wrong things. At the same time, Americans get very little exercise because TVs, computers, smart phones, remotes, cars with power windows, and power toothbrushes—also products we've marketed—have removed the need to exercise at all. So our culture conspires with our economy to create an epidemic of obesity, and with that comes an epidemic of diabetes. And then we celebrate the profits of drug companies and others who make expensive products to treat diabetes, or worse, who manipulate the market to drive up the prices of affordable medications. In a very real sense, the culture of consumer capitalism is our major public health challenge—though try saying *that* on the six o'clock news.

And then, since our culture has created this epidemic of obesity, we spend money on drugs and doctors, instead of spending money on education, housing, public transportation, and the environment—all of which could support and encourage exercise, healthy eating, and locally grown fruits and vegetables that would prevent diabetes if they were eaten instead of industrial produced food-like goop.

Second, we waste at least a trillion dollars a year on health care because we have a health care services market and not a health care system. We haven't asked anyone to create a health care system that has a vision, values, and goals, and there is no one, in government or outside of it, who is held accountable to produce the best health outcomes most affordably.

No one in the United States government with the means and authority to do so is responsible for improving the health of the population. There are a bunch of federal agencies that have limited responsibility for paying for and providing some medical services, and other federal agencies that study the diseases that threaten the health of Americans, and some state and local health departments that have a role in advocating for healthier behaviors (and in protecting the health of the poor). But there is no one organization charged with protecting and improving the health of all of us, so there is no one to hold accountable for our collective failure. Many of the federal agencies are housed within the U.S. Department of Health and Human Services, so we might argue that the DHHS is responsible, but that agency has so many other responsibilities so little actual authority that we can't look to it for leadership.

Inside the DHHS are four agencies concerned with medical services or disease control, each of which has a different purpose.

CMS, the Center for Medicaid and Medicare Services, runs, you guessed it, Medicare and Medicaid. Medicare is a big national insurance plan that pays for health care services for people over sixty-five and people with disabilities, and it has one set of complex rules that apply to all Americans who qualify. Medicaid provides money to each state to pay for health services for the poor, according to certain rules, but each state has to match the federal funding with money raised from state taxes. The Medicaid program for each state works differently, because each state makes some of its own rules. Each state pays hospitals and doctors different amounts for different services, includes or excludes different classes of people, and has a different process for deciding when and how you stay on Medicaid once you qualify for it.

Now get this: some people are eligible for both Medicare and Medicaid. So there are fifty different complicated sets of rules about the people who qualify for both Medicare and Medicaid—and there is a whole special set of bureaucrats who do nothing but write those rules and fight among themselves to figure out how those rules are going to work. Any doctor or hospital that sees a person with both Medicare and Medicaid has to send two separate bills, one to Medicare and the other to Medicaid. Then that doctor or hospital has to track who paid for or didn't pay for what. So we have two sets of folks who write the rules for the two federal programs and state bureaucrats who figure out how to apply those rules and get to write fifty different sets of rules, one set for each state. Then there's another set of folks who try to figure out how all these sets of rules go together, yet others who have to learn those rules, and, of course, the people who generate bills under those rules. But then we need yet another set of folks to check and see if the bills were paid and then argue with Medicare and Medicaid if they weren't. And then there are the people who argue with Congress and state legislatures and the secretary of the DHHS and the president about how much we should pay for what and another set of folks who form national associations of people who want to get paid for stuff or to try to keep us paying for more stuff. And then there are the lawyers . . .

All of these activities are to figure out how to pay for publicly funded health care. But most of the health care that Americans buy is paid for by individuals, private insurance plans, and self-insured employers, each of whom have their own sets of rules about what they pay for and how they pay for it. Which means that there is absolutely no coordination or government oversight of the bulk of the medical services bought and paid for in the U.S. on any given day. CMS may be charged with setting the rules for the insurance that some Americans receive, but it is certainly not in charge of keeping you healthy.

The CDC, the Centers for Disease Control and Prevention, is responsible for the science behind the identification of disease and for designing strategies to prevent, treat, and stop the spread of disease. The CDC has forty thousand scientists and support staff who study emerging diseases and disease patterns and develop ways of keeping disease from spreading. It is a major funder of state departments of health, providing the resources so that those departments can track and prevent the local and regional spread of disease. The CDC doesn't interface much with CMS, which pays for services from private institutions and professionals, often regardless of the public health value of those services. The CDC sometimes sends messages to hospitals and health professionals about what it thinks they should be doing, but those messages take the form of begging, because there are no consequences to hospitals and health professionals for ignoring the CDC, other than the rare malpractice case that references CDC recommendations. State departments of health have real but very limited authority to act in the face of epidemics or in cases of very contagious diseases. They can isolate or even imprison individuals, and they have influence over public schools, deciding what immunizations should be required for school entry, as well as some authority in the case of natural disasters when states of emergency have been declared. But neither the CDC nor state departments of health have the authority or the responsibility to direct any health professional, any hospital or other health care organization to do anything; and neither the CDC nor any state department of health has the responsibility to improve the health of individuals, groups of people living together in one community, or the population as a whole. Both the CDC and state departments of health can report on the health of groups of people and can act in emergency situations, but neither has the resources or the responsibility to change our overall health outcomes.

The Health Resources and Services Administration (HRSA) is responsible for training and deploying different types of health professionals. HRSA also gives grants to help establish and fund community health centers (CHCs). Of all HRSA's work, its role creating and maintaining CHCs is the most important from the perspective of public health. There are 1,375 CHCs in the U.S. that provide primary medical, behavioral health, and dental care to about twenty-five million Americans. CHCs do great work, bringing prevention and medical services to the people who benefit most from those services. That's about one in thirteen Americans—usually people who live in communities where there are economic, geographic, or cultural barriers to health care.

Community health centers are also part of the federal government—sort of. CHCs all receive federal funding through HRSA—start-up funding and about 20 percent of their operational budget. But each CHC is actually an independent nonprofit corporation and is responsible for finding most of its own revenue. CHCs run on money from Medicaid (mostly), Medicare, and private insurance. Most Medicaid revenue is now channeled through private health insurance companies, giving our good friends the insurance companies an extra bite at the public money apple. So while each community health center is directed by HRSA to study and attend to the health of the community in which it is located, CHCs derive most of their income seeing the people who walk through their doors, so that's what they pay most attention to. That means that CHCs focus most on the diseases of the people who come to see them and a little less on *preventing* disease among those people. That also means that CHCs don't spend any time at all on the people in their communities who don't come to see them. Since about 50 percent of people in the U.S. don't seek or get regular primary care, CHCs never get to see or touch half or more than half of the people in the communities they serve.[6] Which means that something like 50 percent of the people in poor communities that otherwise rely on CHCs have no regular medical care, no prevention, no immunizations (unless they are public school children, who have to be immunized in order to attend school), and have no one to see if they get sick, other than the emergency department of the local hospital. Community health centers are great places for the people who use them, but they aren't that effective at improving the measured health outcomes of the communities they serve.[7]

The governance of community health centers is more democratic than the governance of hospitals, but only slightly. Each CHC is its own 501c3 private nonprofit corporation. The good

---

6   We do not know what proportion of the population with a primary care clinician has seen that person for preventative care in the last two years. The CEO of a large insurance company asked this question about his large well-insured population as a favor to me in 2014. Fifty-five percent of that population had a preventative visit in the previous two years. Fifty percent is likely an overestimate of the number of people getting regular prevention in the U.S. Many people use emergency departments and urgent care centers for the bulk of their care.

7   As I write this, the community health center where I worked just turned down a small pot of money from the state department of health, money from the CDC that could have been used to test every patient of the health center for HIV according to the CDC's recommendations. We are in the middle of a HIV outbreak in the community we serve, but the health center only has a limited bandwidth for new programs; the health center's first priority has to be achieving financial stability, so work focused on financial stability always takes priority over public health–oriented programming. This is a very local version of the problem we face as a nation.

news is that each corporation's board must be 51 percent patients. The bad news is that those board members are appointed by the existing board members (and usually nominated by the existing executive director), instead of being elected by members of the community or users of the community health center. That means boards of CHCs often do not reflect the racial, cultural, and social class composition of the communities they serve. It also means the executive leadership and the boards themselves often develop the same kind of cozy relationship that hospital boards have with their executive leadership, and that sometimes decisions get made that have less to do with the health care needs of the communities CHCs serve and more to do with making sure that executive leadership keeps itself employed and in control.

The CHCs don't constitute a true health care system with a single mission, vision, values, and goals for the poor. Instead, there is only a patchwork of very good health centers, some weaker and others stronger, which depend on community boards and executive directors to set policy and deliver the services critical to the protection of our most vulnerable people. The CDC has no influence over community health centers, so the CDC has to beg CHCs to pay attention to the public's health, as it does with hospitals and health professionals. CMS has no control of community health centers either. CHCs are just another seller of health services from the CMS perspective, although, as you may have guessed, there is a special set of CMS rules about how Medicare and Medicaid pay health centers.

And then there is the SAMHSA, the Substance Abuse and Mental Health Services Administration, which provides expert information about substance abuse and mental health services and funds drug treatment programs and community mental health centers (which are different from community health centers). It's a completely different bureaucracy from HRSA, with different rules, different grant programs, different beliefs, and different practices. Which means, at the local level, the community health center doesn't usually talk to the community mental health center, which doesn't talk to drug treatment programs, most of which are private and many of which are for-profit.

Then there is the Food and Drug Administration, the FDA. The FDA also lives at the Department of Health and Human Services. It regulates pharmaceutical and medical device manufacturers to make sure the products they manufacture are safe, and it regulates food and food products. That's the good news. The bad news is that the FDA operates under authorizing legislation passed by Congress and depends on funding from Congress provided in yearly appropriations. Congress responds to the needs and wants of special interests, which include drug and pharmaceutical manufacturers, large industrial food producers, and others in the agricultural industry—the very same companies that the FDA is regulating. And because too few Americans vote, there is little to balance the needs of those interests when Congress deliberates and passes authorizing legislation and the yearly budget. Which means the FDA, as pure and disinterested as it wants to make itself out to be, is always swayed by the needs of special interests and creates a host of compromises and special opportunities, which Congress approves at the behest of those special interests, at the end of the day. Those compromises allow pharmaceutical companies to have inappropriate monopolies on drugs that they didn't actually develop and to market old drugs with new "delivery systems," permitting them to overprice drugs that are no different from those that have been in the market for years. These compromises have slowed the development of food labeling, so food labels don't reflect what is actually healthy and don't make sense to normal folk. These compromises have also prevented us from developing realistic cigarette and tobacco labeling, given that tobacco is a hundred times more dangerous than most people understand.

Finally, there is the U.S. Department of Agriculture (USDA), which provides subsidies to farmers and runs both the Food Stamp Program (formally, the Supplemental Nutrition Assistance Program, or SNAP, in case you need one more acronym for your collection). Now, if you think that the USDA isn't part of the health care enterprise, think again. The foods people eat have a major impact on their health, but the USDA isn't empowered to protect health. It is responsible for helping farmers, promoting agriculture, and stimulating American farmers and farm product-based conglomerates to produce and sell more stuff, regardless of how healthy—or dangerous—that stuff is. And because existing corporate interests have very powerful lobbyists, the programs initially established to help small farmers survive have become expensive corporate welfare projects that are exceedingly hard to change, because those focused interests know just how to play our sometimes unbalanced representative democracy, which gives a lot of Senate votes to farm states.[8]

So we subsidize corn, wheat, sugar, beef, and hogs, which means that we produce more corn, wheat, sugar, beef, and hogs than we can eat. We produce so much corn that producers have to make lots of very cheap high-fructose corn syrup to use up some of the excess—it is that cheap sweetener that is added to industrially produced and mass marketed food-like products and that helped trigger the epidemic of diabetes and obesity now sweeping the county. Think about what our nation would look like if we subsidized apples, carrots, celery, lettuce, watermelon, and beets, for example. If fruits and vegetables were cheaper than tap water, and if industrially produced food-like goop cost

---

8   The political career of Senator George McGovern ended after he chaired the Senate Select Committee on Nutrition and Human Needs and that committee recommended that Americans eat (a little) less beef. The beef lobby went after him, and he lost his next—and last—election.

an arm and a leg. Some people want us to tax sugar-sweetened beverages as a way to slow their consumption, because those beverages have been associated with the epidemic of obesity and diabetes. Wouldn't it be cheaper and easier to make sugar and high-fructose corn syrup expensive to grow and produce in the first place and to subsidize healthy foods? The USDA could use subsidies if it were a health agency. But the USDA is a corporate pawn, a government agency that has helped produce an epidemic while creating profit for a few corporations.

When I was in government in Rhode Island, I fought hard for food stamp use to be restricted to safe and healthy foods and brought the case for that restriction to the highest levels of the USDA. I was told: good idea but not politically possible. That is to say, everyone at the USDA understood that their policy was crazy, but they knew that Congress would never let them change the policy because of the power of lobbyists for corporate food producers and senators from the farm states. And that was during the Obama administration, during the heyday of the Tea Party, so you'd think progressives who like the idea of science-based regulation ought to be able to join with the people who hate all expensive government programs to reform an expensive government program that was off the tracks. But no dice. The dark side of the force was still too powerful.

And that's only the chaos inside government. The chaos in the private sector is worse.

There are about 5,600 hospitals in the U.S. About 20 percent of them are for-profit. The state, local, or federal government owns another 20 percent. The rest—60 percent of our hospitals—are private nonprofit hospitals, which means they are technically independent of everyone and have governing boards made up of community leaders, who in theory make sure that each hospital does what the community needs. *In theory*.

We spend about a trillion dollars a year on hospitals, or about 32 percent of all our spending on health care.[9] Most of our spending on hospitals—60 to 65 percent—is public funds from Medicare and Medicaid. About 25 percent of that public spending by Medicare and Medicaid—$150-250 billion a year—is spent on administrative overhead, not on patient care. Most nonprofit hospitals (about 60 percent of all hospitals) are private not-for-profit corporations, which means they don't pay taxes on their earnings, even though they pay their senior executives millions of dollars a year. Most nonprofit hospitals have volunteer boards of directors, but most boards are nominated by their executives (the ones who are paid millions of dollars a year) and appointed by the existing boards, not elected by either their patients or the communities they serve.

So we have this patchwork of hospitals that serve the people who come through their doors but are not required by anyone to perform specific functions for specific communities. They exist on public funds but have no public accountability, other than some state licensing requirements, which require only that each hospital isn't committing terrible errors like wrong-site surgery or running hospital-acquired infection rates that are worse than those of other hospitals. No one requires hospitals to have the best achievable infection rates. Hospitals are only required to have infection rates that aren't too much worse than the rates at other hospitals, because if any regulator gets too strict, the hospital association sends their lobbyists to complain to the governor and the legislature, who then cut off the regulator's funding unless the regulator backs down.

---

9   Centers for Medicare and Medicaid Services, "National Health Expenditures 2016 Highlights," available at https://www.cms.gov/Research-Statistics-Data-and-Systems/Statistics-Trends-and-Reports/NationalHealthExpendData/downloads/highlights.pdf (accessed April 28, 2018).

Hospitals pay their senior executives millions of dollars, which come from public funds, and spend 25 percent of their revenue (again, mostly public funds) on bureaucracy, not patient care. (The for-profit hospitals sometimes spend less on administration, but they often pay their executives even higher salaries and take more money out of the health care budget as profit for investors.) And all these hospitals compete with one another for patients. That means hospitals try their level best to hospitalize more people and do more tests and procedures—regardless of the actual health impact of those tests and procedures—because that is how they make the money they need to survive as business entities. Remember, hospitals have no responsibility for improving or protecting the public's health. Their job is only to stay in business and not get caught killing anyone.

Is this a health care system or a kleptocracy?

Now, say we were to try to reorganize hospitals and hospital boards in the U.S. Do you think for one second that the political system would let us do that? Every lobbyist in America would descend on Congress and on our state legislatures. They would use every trick in the book to keep these publicly funded hospitals from becoming accountable for improving the public's health. Yet public funds are the source of the hospital income that is used to employ the lobbyists, who do everything they can to make sure hospitals are better paid—and remain accountable to no one.

State departments of health regulate hospitals and other health care institutions, monitor the health status of the population of states, respond to threats faced by those populations, help protect the safety of food, water, and air, work to keep infectious diseases in check, and support states responding to health emergencies. Most of the funding for departments of health comes from the CDC, and most state departments are good at providing the public with information about health risks and ways to prevent those risks. But, with the exception of some local offices that target immunizing the children of the very poor, state departments of health usually don't have any boots on the ground. They don't have ways to touch individuals who may be ill, only procedures to identify people at risk and then refer them to hospitals and health professionals for treatment. State departments of health also have to do a fair amount of begging and always have to approach any regulation gingerly. They have to beg hospitals, nursing homes, and health professionals to use safe practices, because the departments are only empowered to close down operations that are manifestly unsafe. Departments don't have any way to ensure that health care institutions focus on best practices and the public's health and must be very careful about how much they regulate because of political considerations that they have to live with as governmental entities. If those departments dare to say that guns kill people, point out that the sale of alcohol may be associated with drug and alcohol overdose deaths, or to suggest that the sale of sugar-sweetened beverages is associated with obesity, then the lobbyists for those "industries" descend on the legislature, and the legislature may take away the budgets of the departments of health. So departments are exceptionally cautious about what they say about dangerous products because of who they might offend, and because they want to make sure that the other critical public health work they do can continue.

Boards of professional licensure and discipline, national boards of medical examiners, and specialty certification boards exist to make sure that health professionals practice their professions ethically and responsibly. These boards try to prevent health professionals from hurting the public as they pursue their professions, and, even more, they work to create public confidence in the health professions—so that when a patient dies in a dental chair, people don't quit going to dentists because the public assumes that all dentists are dangerous, or when an anesthesiologist sexually abuses a woman under anesthesia, people don't quit getting surgery because they are afraid of all anesthesiologists. These boards have a protective role but not a health promotional role. Their existence recognizes that health professionals without regulation pose a risk to the public. Most of these boards are heavily influenced by the health sector's professional organizations, and many are housed in other parts of state government—in departments of commerce or insurance regulation—instead of inside state departments of health, so in many states there is absolutely no linkage between what health professionals do and any public health goals or objectives. Most board members are political appointees and, given the influence wielded by these professional organizations' lobbyists, most can be undermined or destroyed by state legislatures should they ever become too proactive.

Health professionals—doctors, dentists, and nurses, among others—are private businesspeople, who earn a living by selling their services. Health professionals are not charged with any public function at all. Professionals either practice on their own or are employees. Their only real obligation is to do no harm and to provide the advice and care that they give without regard to self-interest—that is, to give the correct advice based on science and professional standards and not give advice that would benefit themselves instead of the patients they care for. That's a pretty low bar. No health professional is required to do any affirmative good. Some of us hope that health professionals recognize an ethical imperative to advocate for better social conditions when the science tells us that social conditions are the cause of people's illness, but that advocacy is voluntary and difficult given the work lives of health professionals and the social pressure not to criticize things as they are.

Health insurance companies provide people personal financial protection in case of illness or injury. American businesses and individuals spent about $1.1 trillion on private health insurance in 2014—about $1.3-1.4 trillion by the time you read this.[10] Insurers are just like Medicare—they pay for services that the people they cover purchase. Health insurance companies themselves retain between 10 and 20 percent of the dollars they collect and use that money for overhead, administrative cost, salaries, and profit—that's $150-300 billion a year. They have no business interest in the health of the population, and they have little business interest in providing health care at the lowest possible cost. Their only job is to compete with one another. That means each health insurance company wants to drive costs down a little—but only enough to attract more business than their competition. Insurers use their market power—their ability to direct more business to doctors and hospitals—to demand lower prices. But if insurers drive the cost down too much, they risk alienating the people they are paying—doctors and hospitals—who can leverage their relationships with patients and the community to shift business away from the insurer who is low-cost. That means the largest hospitals, specialty groups, and drug companies—market actors with the most market power who have close to a monopoly on a specific service—can best resist the power of insurers. So when insurers try to drive down costs, the weakest sectors—usually, primary care doctors and community health centers—absorb most of spending reductions because they don't have the market power or the lobbying muscle they need to fight back. That's because primary care doctors and community health centers focus their efforts on public health, community needs, and the needs of the patients they serve, instead of merging to jockey for market leverage.

But the insurance process itself increases overall health care cost, even as insurers try to reduce the cost of each purchased health service. Because insurers focus on the cost of each service

---

10 "National Health Expenditures and Percent Distribution, by Sponsor: United States, Selected Years 1987-2014," available at http://www.cdc.gov/nchs/data/hus/2015/100.pdf (accessed April 13, 2018).

and not the cost of keeping people healthy, other market actors—doctors, hospitals, pharmaceutical companies, and medical device manufacturers—use the market to sell more services so that they can make more money, even as insurers try to cut the cost of each service a little bit. That's why you see billboards near the highway advertising the emergency room of the local hospital, and that's why you see commercials on television promoting those cool little scooters people with disabilities drive. Health care providers and businesses are better at increasing utilization than insurers are at reducing the cost of each service. We know that because health care cost keeps increasing at about 3 to 6 percent or more a year—twice the rate of inflation. Insurance is like a blank check, an open credit card for anyone who has it, and people with something to sell realize they can sell more of what they make or do to people with insurance by advertising a lot.

If you are a drug company and the mean insurance company will only pay one hundred dollars for your drug, you can just go out and convince a zillion more people that they need your drug, whether the drug has real benefit or not, and you'll make more money, despite what the insurance company pays for each one. If you are a gastroenterologist, a doctor who sells colonoscopies, you just go out and convince a zillion more people to have a colonoscopy, thereby protecting or increasing your income, regardless of what the insurance company decides to pay you, and regardless of whether colonoscopies protect or improve the public health. (Some do. Many don't.)

Notice that none of this buying and selling and paying for has any direct relationship to protecting the public's health. Sometimes, some people get medical services they actually need, but that's by accident, not design.

From the perspective of public health, it is community health centers, primary care doctors, and primary care practices that have the most value. They focus on prevention and they provide inexpensive access to health professionals who aren't trying to sell the public something. But there is nothing about the insurance process that causes insurers to pay for that value, and there is no incentive whatsoever for health insurers to fund a system of primary care practices and community health centers to provide affordable health care to all Americans.

There is a mountain of evidence that shows how access to primary care improves public health outcomes and reduces cost. Remember that health insurance companies consume 10 to 20 percent of what we spend on health care just to pay for the insurance process alone, while primary care doctors and practices and community health centers consume only about 5 percent of the entire health care budget—or about one-quarter to one-half of what insurance overhead consumes. For what it costs us just to run the damn insurance companies, we could give primary care to all Americans, in their own communities, in health centers that are open from 8:00 a.m. to 8:00 p.m. and on weekends. Instead, we enact reforms that bring insurance companies more and more money.

Health insurance may turn out to injure the public's health at the end of the day. The health insurance process causes us to buy and sell many medical procedures and products that are actually harmful, especially when used unnecessarily—something like a trillion dollars worth of what's unnecessary. The health insurance process and the market it has created reduces the amount of money that federal, state, and local governments and individuals have to spend on other programs and products— such as better housing, better education, better public transportation, and community development—that have been shown to improve the public's health. The health insurance process allows the consolidation of more and more money, providing money for insurers, hospitals, pharmaceutical companies, doctors, and device manufacturers to lobby Congress, state governments, and regulatory agencies, strengthening their own positions, while weakening the democratic process and steering funding further away from the programs and purchases that actually matter for health. The health insurance process enriches executives and shareholders of health insurance companies, hospitals, pharmaceutical companies, device manufacturers, and health professionals, increasing the gap between rich and poor, a gap that weakens democracy and that some public health experts believe is in itself associated with poor public health outcomes.

And what happens to our democracy in this process? Insurance companies, their trade organizations, and their lobbyists were at the center of the health insurance reform of 2009 and 2010—and they made out like bandits. They got $110-120 billion of new business. All the rest of us got more debt, no clear evidence of improved health status, more political polarization, and more income inequality. Twenty million of us got health insurance. History will determine if that was a good thing.

Look around. We've been sold a bill of goods.

The third reason our health care market costs so much but produces poor health outcomes is that we let people profit by selling products that are dangerous. Alcohol, firearms, industrially produced food-like goop, television, tobacco—you name it. If there is something that injures the public's health but makes someone some money, you can be sure there is a trade group promoting it and a host of lobbyists making sure there is no impediment to selling it to anyone with a dollar, despite what those products cost the public in terms of lost life, lost productivity, lost wages, and public dollars for medical care to address the health problems that all those products cause.

We sell industrial food-like products that can only make you sick. We sell alcohol and advertise drugs as the solution to all life's problems. Then we are shocked, shocked when lots of people start taking these drugs and a host of others, like the advertisements on TV and on billboards and on the internet tell them to do. We sell guns—250 to 360 million at last count—and then we are shocked, shocked when people use them on each other. Because guns don't kill people, only people kill people. We sell labor-saving devices, so you don't have to leave your chair to change the channel, and there is a button to roll down the window, and another button that will brush your teeth, and then we are shocked, shocked when Americans become obese and get diabetes because they aren't getting enough exercise.

The fourth way we generate unnecessary health care cost and create poor health outcomes is that we allow people to live in poverty and to live with racism, which keeps the health of some of us unnecessarily poor. Poverty and racism make the people who experience them sick from the stress of living that way and from living in places that the rest of us have abandoned because they are so dangerous.[11]

The fifth way we allow too much health care cost and accept poor outcomes is that we don't fund or promote government's

---

11 Conservative pundits tend to blame the poor performance of our health care market on race, arguing that our health care market only appears to perform poorly because it has to care for so many (African American and Latino) people who are so much sicker than white people, and their numbers cloud the intrinsic effectiveness of the market. This argument is a new kind of racism, in its way. There is nothing about skin color in America that predicts high infant mortality or reduced life expectancy, because there is only the weakest association between skin color and genetics, if there is an association at all. If our market was effective it would be able to improve the health of all Americans regardless of race and to do that equally. But skin color predicts how some Americans are treated by our culture, and that treatment is what predicts infant mortality and life expectancy. To blame the poor outcomes achieved by our health care market on the diversity of our population is to blame the victims of discrimination twice—once, for suffering the discrimination that causes the poor outcomes, and a second time for "causing" our health care market to have the appearance of poor outcomes because our population is diverse, even though all those poor outcomes were caused by racism in the first place.

role in promoting health. Federal, state, and local governments could be much more effective as regulators of health professionals and health care institutions and as guardians of the public purse, making sure we get public value from public spending. But not enough of us vote, so there is no one making sure that our government delivers what it promises and no one to make government accountable to the people it serves, instead of bending over for lobbyists and stakeholders looking only to protect their own incomes.

Finally, the most profound way we allow too much health care cost and accept poor outcomes is that we have allowed a health care market to masquerade as a health care system. The United States has no health care system that provides the same set of necessary services to all Americans. There is no one in government who is responsible for making sure everyone is immunized or responsible for making sure everyone over fifty who actually needs a colonoscopy gets one, or that everyone is tested for HIV and hepatitis C. If we had a health care system that touched all Americans and that brought all Americans prevention where we live and medical services that are appropriate to the injuries and illness that we have, instead of being scaled to the profit aspirations investors have, we would be able to improve the health of all and reduce the cost by a trillion dollars a year or more. Think that wealth might be put to work in other ways? A trillion dollars buys a lot of education, safe and healthy housing, public transportation, and environmental improvement—and maybe even new leisure time so that we might all enjoy each other and our own lives more.

We pay for the health care market as we know it three times over. It costs us an extra trillion dollars a year. It worsens the measurable health of our population. And it weakens our democracy.

We can do better than this.

CHAPTER TWO

We Have a Market, Not a Health Care System

IN AUGUST 2012, JENNIFER MILLER, WHO LIVES IN WESTFIELD, NEW JERSEY, took her daughter Caroline into Manhattan for Caroline's yearly checkup, just in time for her to start kindergarten. Caroline's amazing pediatrician recommended a flu shot, something Caroline got every year, but the flu shots weren't available yet at her pediatrician's office. I'll get my kids the shots in the fall, Jennifer told herself, as soon as they become available. Maybe at a walk-in, because that's easier than driving into the city. She might have seen signs in front of CVS stores advertising flu vaccine, because in 2012 CVS had obtained a supply of vaccine and was advertising it heavily by August, but Jennifer doesn't remember those signs now.

It was a busy fall. Caroline started full-day kindergarten. She had swimming lessons and gymnastics lessons and playdates, and Jennifer, running from place to place, forgot to call her pediatrician or go to a walk-in October.

The flu vaccine just wasn't such a big deal in 2012. Influenza seemed like a pretty routine illness, much like the common cold, one of those diseases you could prevent with vaccine if you wanted to, but it didn't matter all that much. Jennifer's own doctor never pushed her to get a flu shot. Jennifer doesn't remember whether her pediatrician's office, as good as they were, called to remind her to get Caroline a flu shot after the vaccine came in, usually in mid-October. Perhaps they did. Perhaps not.

Then it was Halloween, then it was Thanksgiving, and then there was the holiday rush. Jennifer meant to get Caroline the shot. The idea of taking Caroline to CVS for the shot never really crossed Jennifer's mind. CVS was for people who didn't have a doctor, and New Jersey didn't let pharmacists give children shots anyway.

Then on December 18, just four days after the murders of those schoolchildren in Sandy Hook, Caroline came home with a cold. She had a runny nose and a cough, which worsened as the evening progressed, and Jennifer called the pediatrician. Caroline had mild asthma and used medications to control it, so the pediatrician told told Jennifer to start the asthma medicine. But Caroline's breathing got worse. Jennifer called the pediatrician back, and he, a great diagnostician indeed, asked Jennifer to put Caroline on the phone. Over the phone, by listening to the cadence of her breathing, the pediatrician recognized the seriousness of Caroline's breathing problem and told Jennifer to get her to the nearest hospital right away, even though it was the middle of the night.

Overlook Hospital, in Summit, New Jersey, is a very good community hospital. They immediately diagnosed influenza A—and pneumonia—and started Caroline on medicine and oxygen. And, as sick as she was, Caroline looked okay. She was alert and playful. Her color was good. Jennifer assumed Caroline would get medicine for a day or two, perhaps stay in the hospital for a few days, but would be home in plenty of time for Christmas.

But Caroline's breathing and general condition worsened. Caroline stopped acting like herself. She had no color in her face. Her hands were cool and clammy. Jennifer got scared. The doctors at Overlook decided to transfer Caroline by ambulance to Morristown Hospital, about ten miles away, where there was a pediatric intensive care unit, and the ambulance ran to Morristown hot, with Caroline getting oxygen the whole time, lights and sirens all the way.

The doctors at Morristown took one look at Caroline and decided to intubate her and put her on a ventilator. Then they started talking about moving Caroline to yet another hospital, one that had special support for kids who had what doctors call respiratory failure, kids whose lungs aren't working at all. Jennifer was frightened, but she was having trouble keeping up with events because they were moving so fast. Caroline was really sick, that was clear, but it was hard to believe she needed to be so far from home. The doctors were talking about hospitals in New York and Philadelphia and about helicopters. They were trying to decide whether to send her right then or wait until morning and see if they could get Caroline stabilized. Jennifer wasn't sure what to do. She didn't want her daughter to be so far from home.

At that moment, Caroline's pediatrician did what few other doctors anywhere in the county would have done. He walked into Morristown Hospital, a hospital thirty miles from his office, where he didn't have admitting privileges and didn't know any of the staff. He looked at Caroline, looked at Jennifer, and said, "Why wait? Let's move her now."

Caroline was moved by helicopter to the Children's Hospital of Philadelphia, one of the most sophisticated children's hospitals in the nation. She spent two weeks at death's door but somehow she survived. She had a stormy four-week hospital course, including two weeks in the Pediatric Intensive Care Unit, where she was treated for pneumonia, acute respiratory distress syndrome, sepsis, and septic shock. She came home two weeks after New Year's Day and normal life returned.

Too many other children like her aren't so lucky. Too many American kids don't get immunized against the flu. About one hundred children die of influenza each year in the U.S. Most of them are poor kids of color, and most weren't immunized against influenza.[1]

1 Brendan Flannery et al. "Influenza Vaccine Effectiveness Against Pediatric Deaths: 2010-2014," *Pediatrics* 139, no. 5 (April 2017), available at http://pediatrics.aappublications.org/content/early/2017/03/30/peds.2016-4244 (accessed April 20, 2018).

Caroline is a child who lives in a suburb. She has two great parents who can afford health insurance, a great pediatrician, swimming and gymnastics lessons—parents who have the time to drive her to playdates. They had a doctor they could call when Caroline got sicker. They had a car to put her in to drive her to the hospital in the middle of the night. And they were the kind of people who knew how to make sure that their child was going by helicopter to the best children's hospital in the nation when Caroline got sicker yet.

Few American kids are that lucky. Few American kids have doctors as good as her pediatrician or have access to hospitals as good as Overlook, Morristown Hospital, and the Children's Hospital of Philadelphia, organized coherently so that is it easy to move a sick child from one to the next when needed.

Even fewer American kids have pediatricians or community health centers who know each child and who can bug parents until each child gets a flu shot every year. The families of some kids are reminded about the flu vaccine, but not every kid, not by far, which is why only 60 percent of American children are vaccinated against influenza each year in the U.S. We do a better job immunizing kids against flu than we do immunizing adults. We do a better job with kids because we have a school system that requires all our kids to be in school, and to be in school every child is *supposed* to be immunized. But we have no system to *get* every American child immunized.[2]

In the U.S., we have about thirty thousand unnecessary deaths a year from influenza—deaths from influenza and from the pneumonia that influenza often causes in the very young and

---

2   Every kid goes to school, and the rules about vaccination for school entry—and our *system* of school nurse teachers in every school—makes sure every kid is vaccinated against most childhood diseases. But the school vaccination system doesn't work for influenza vaccine, because few schools require influenza vaccination for school attendance, the way other vaccines are required.

in people with other health problems—thirty thousand deaths that might have been prevented if everyone in the country got a flu shot each fall. We argue about the efficacy of the vaccine, which varies from year to year, and about the extent to which the claim of thirty thousand deaths is inflated by pharma and immunization advocates, because that number includes all deaths caused by pneumonia and influenza, many of which would not be prevented by the vaccine. But truth be told, we've never had a good test of the effectiveness of the vaccine because our influenza vaccination rate is so poor. Right now, about 43 percent of adults and 60 percent of children get immunized, while 57 percent of adults, and 40 percent of children—about 170 million people—don't.

Here's what we do now to get people immunized. First the CDC, in partnership with the World Health Organization, figures out how to create a vaccine for the epidemic we think is coming.[3] Using the CDC's instructions, pharmaceutical companies begin producing the vaccine in the spring of each year for fall shipment, a process licensed and overseen by the FDA. The CDC predicts how many doses we'll need, and it buys a few million doses for a certain subset of children and adults who are most vulnerable. Pharmaceutical companies decide how much flu vaccine to produce based on how much they think they can sell. Clinicians, hospitals, state and local health departments, mass immunizers, home health agencies, and pharmaceutical retailers make separate deals for vaccine, which is why CVS

---

3 The influenza vaccine is usually assembled from three or four different vaccines that protect people against the strains of virus most likely to be causing disease in the coming year. Since the annual influenza epidemic usually moves from west to east, the disease in circulation in China in one year typically becomes the virus in circulation in the U.S. the following fall. So we base our predictions on strains of virus that are making people and animals sick in other parts of the world—usually in China and other parts of Asia.

had the vaccine before Caroline's pediatrician did, and then they all try to talk people into getting the vaccine. Clinicians, hospitals, pharmaceutical retailers, home health agencies, and mass immunizers administer the vaccine. Then CMS pays for the vaccine for people it insures using at least three different processes—one for Medicare, a different one for Medicaid, and a third process for community health centers. Private health insurance companies, individuals, and employers pay for the rest. The CDC distributes the doses it buys to state departments of health, who give those doses to local departments of health, hospitals, community health centers, and private physicians for administration to a subset of the population. The people who administer the CDC's purchased doses don't charge for the vaccine itself, but they do charge somebody—usually Medicare or Medicaid but sometimes private insurers—for the administration of the vaccine.[4]

So for the flu vaccine we have lots of market actors—pharmaceutical companies, insurance companies, retail pharmacies, hospitals, visiting nurse associations, primary care clinicians, vaccine administration organizations, and a number of government agencies—all participating in a process that gives us a flu vaccination rate of between 40 and 60 percent, depending on age. But no one counts the number of people who still need vaccinating each fall, and no one is out there calling the people who haven't been vaccinated yet or taking vaccine to their homes,

---

4 This process has turned flu vaccine into a commodity that is bought and sold like sugar, beets, or oil, with its own futures market and brokers. Vaccinators have to rebook vaccine orders in January and February for the coming year, guessing how much vaccine they will need the following year, if they are to get any supply at all. In heavy flu seasons, when people get sicker than usual from the flu, or in years the flu vaccine manufacturers encounter technical problems in producing the vaccine, we see shortages of vaccine, and then there emerges a spot market for the vaccine, with the price of any spare job lots of vaccine shooting up in cost, sometimes going for twice what the vaccine usually costs.

workplaces, or places of worship. No one is pushing vaccine manufacturers to make all the vaccine we need instead of only making the vaccine we think we can sell.

Vaccinating 40 to 60 percent of the population isn't terrible but is not enough to achieve something called herd immunity, which happens when so many people are immunized that disease doesn't spread in the population. That is what we need to achieve if we are to avoid most preventable deaths from influenza and pneumonia. Now imagine another approach. Let's say that we had a Ministry of Health that had a budget from the federal government, and that our ministry used its budget to buy vaccine in bulk for all the people in the U.S. every year. Let us also imagine that every community had a local health center that was open from eight in the morning to eight at night and on weekends. Let's imagine that these health centers provided primary care, mental health care, and substance abuse treatment and were charged with immunizing everyone in the city or town in which they were located, for which they were paid. So, in addition to immunizing people in clinics at health centers, they might also immunize people in schools, in supermarkets, in shopping plazas, at the polls on election day, in bars, in barbershops, in churches, mosques, and synagogues— wherever people congregate. Suppose that health centers kept track of everyone they had and had not immunized. These centers might well call each unimmunized person to remind them and even bring the vaccine to that person's house. Suppose someone had noticed in November that Caroline hadn't been immunized and had brought the vaccine to her house or school. Caroline probably would not have gotten sick.

If we got rid of all the intermediaries—the people who buy and sell vaccine and the people who send bills and pay the bills for every person who gets vaccinated—don't you think we could immunize more people at a lower cost? Don't you think we could get the immunization rate to 90 percent or even higher?

And don't you think we could save the lives of the hundred kids or more who die of influenza each year, the bulk of whom are poor or of color and missed their flu shot that year?

Consider HIV and hepatitis C for a moment—both are treatable diseases that we have failed to control appropriately because we don't have a health care system. And notice who gains and who loses because of how we do health care in the U.S.

Each new person who gets HIV generates about $400,000 in lifetime health care costs, of which 75 percent is for medications.[5] Most of these costs are paid out of tax revenue, because most people with HIV and AIDS have Medicaid or Medicare. So every new infection we don't prevent costs a lot of money, and of course every infection that goes undiagnosed causes untold human suffering and too many unnecessary deaths. If we had a health care system and had stopped HIV transmission in, say, 2000, then we'd have far fewer people living with HIV and far fewer needing expensive drugs. Assuming that we have seen about 40,000 new cases of HIV diagnoses a year since 2000, that means about 680,000 of the 1.2 million people now living with HIV or AIDS have been diagnosed since 2000.[6] If the treatment of each person costs about $20,000 a year, then we are spending about $13.6 billion a year on treatment of a disease that was preventable, to say nothing of the suffering each of those 680,000 people experienced unnecessarily. But there is a flip side to this cost. If we are spending $13.6 billion we didn't need to spend, some pharmaceutical company is making $13.6 billion that it shouldn't

5   Bruce R. Schackman et al. "The Lifetime Medical Cost Savings from Preventing HIV in the United States," *Medical Care* 53, no. 4 (April 2015): 293–301, available at https://www.ncbi.nlm.nih.gov/pubmed/25710311 (accessed April 13, 2018).

6   Centers for Disease Control and Prevention, "HIV in the Unites States: *At a Glance*," available at https://www.cdc.gov/hiv/statistics/overview/ ataglance.html (accessed April 13, 2018).

be making. That means not having a health care system is costing us $13.6 billion a year in HIV treatment a year alone. This $13.6 billion ends up in the coffers of pharmaceutical companies and others who profit when we fail to address a preventable disease, rather than being spent on education, housing, the environment, and public safety, which turn out to be what matters if we are going to improve the public's health.

The moral quandary we face is that for every person who gets a disease that could have been prevented if we had a health care system, some other person makes a pretty good living by selling a treatment or a cure, while some essential service goes unfunded.

It is worth noting that pharmaceutical companies had a major role in developing effective HIV drugs, and they would argue that their profit is justified by the risk they take to develop new medications. Pharmaceutical companies take risk when they invest in research and development, when they test the drugs they've developed, and when they have to steer their new drugs through the FDA's lengthy and expensive regulatory process. Few of the drugs that are developed in the lab make it to market, they would say, and they have to bear the costs of the whole process of trial and error and of an intense regulatory process, and no one in their right mind would engage in drug development if there wasn't a substantial reward for success.

We too often forget that government also had a substantial role in the development of HIV drugs, as it did in the development of hepatitis C drugs. Government entities—the NIH and the CDC—organized research attention around both HIV and hepatitis C, which I'll discuss in more detail later. Public funds are used for the foundational research and often for early clinical trials. But when it comes time to bring these drugs to market, only the private sector reaps the profits. Some argue that the private sector achieved what government and academia could never have achieved—to be able to treat these two difficult infectious diseases in short order. But it is still not clear why more of the return on the initial investments in research that supported much of the basic science and other research that led to these miracle treatments doesn't come back to the public.

And it turns out the government pays for most of these drugs. At least 40 percent of people being treated for HIV or AIDS have Medicaid, another 20 percent have Medicare, and more than 10 percent have both.[7] In 2018, the federal government is expected to pay out $26 billion for HIV care, and state governments are likely to pay $3-4 billion—close to $30 billion of public funding for HIV care—the bulk of which is for medications.[8] (The $13.6 billion discussed in the thought experiment on pages 40-41 is a little less than half that amount, which makes sense because it represents the cost of care for more than half of the total HIV population—the number of infections that could have been prevented if we'd had a way to screen the entire population in the year 2000. But $13.6 million is likely an *underestimate* of the extra spending on HIV/AIDS that resulted from our inability to test all Americans aged thirteen to sixty-four in 2000, because it includes the cost of drugs paid for by private insurers. And that number completely fails to capture the human tragedy

---

7 "Medicaid and HIV," *KFF*, October 14, 2016, available at https://www.kff.org/hivaids/fact-sheet/medicaid-and-hiv/ (accessed May 17, 2018).

8 "Federal Domestic HIV/AIDS Programs & Research Spending," *HIV.gov*, January 18, 2018, available at https://www.hiv.gov/federal-response/funding/budget (accessed May 17, 2018). The state Medicaid spend is an estimate, based on the federal Medicaid spend in 2018, which was budgeted at $6.1 billion. Medicaid is a 50/50 match of state to federal funds, except for people who enrolled in Medicaid as a result of the Affordable Care Act. The federal government is responsible for 100 percent of the costs for that group. "U.S. Federal Funding for HIV/AIDS: Trends Over Time," *KFF*, January, November 9, 2017, available at https://www.kff.org/global-health-policy/fact-sheet/u-s-federal-funding-for-hivaids-trends-over-time/ (accessed May 17, 2018).

represented by the 680,000 people whose HIV could have been prevented.)

We have created a situation in which we used public money to do foundational research for drug development, handed that research over to private corporations to complete the development, and then paid private corporations high prices for the drugs themselves, allowing those corporations to reap huge profits, the bulk of which come from public funds.

Our approach to drug development and drug pricing poses questions about what is appropriate and what is fair, what should be public and what private, how much profit is appropriate, and what we lose by allowing so much profit for drugs that are developed by pharma. Clearly, we spend more public money then we need to in this process, but we lose something else when we move public resources into private pockets. The transfer of wealth from public control to private control means that we have fewer public resources to use to build our public infrastructure— our schools and our public housing and our community centers and our public transportation—and so everyone suffers. This transfer of wealth also means that pharma has more money to spend on lobbying, which leads to the transfer of more public money to pharma over time.

But it doesn't have to be this way. We ought to be able have government itself handle drug development and keep the patent rights, contracting out only drug manufacture, so we could keep profits low. Or we could set prices for drugs, allowing a small profit margin but not a profit margin that is astronomical. Or we could give government an equity stake in drug development that was built on government-funded foundational research, so some of the profits return to the public pocketbook. At the end of the day, when we allow ungodly profit for medicines, we lose in two ways—we create an inhuman obstacle for people who are ill, who fear for their lives because of the cost of the medication, and we undermine the possibility of full democracy, because we give some of us the means to influence government that others lack.

Hepatitis C became a more common cause of death than HIV in 2008 while everyone's head was turned away. The availability of treatment for hepatitis C represents both a huge success of drug development and another story about how we weaken democracy because we have a health care market instead of a health care system.

Hepatitis C was isolated in 1989 by researchers at the Chiron Corporation, which was started by three academics at the University of California who had been trained and paid with public funds. These three researchers began collaborating with researchers at the CDC and the NIH and were able to isolate the cause of what was then known as non-A-non-B hepatitis.[9] Hepatitis C is transmitted through blood products, through sexual contact, sometimes by household contact, and occasionally by needles used by tattoo artists, acupuncturists, and dentists who haven't employed proper infection control in their practices. Most hepatitis C spread came from needle sharing by people who were using drugs in the late 1960s and early 1970s, and who then donated or sold their blood to blood banks, which supplied the tainted blood to hospitals and kidney dialysis centers for transfusion. Chiron created a blood test for hepatitis C shortly after isolating the virus, and that test came into wide use in 1992, at which point the blood supply stopped being a major route of transmission. Transmission today is mostly among people who share needles or are sexually active with an infected

---

9   The isolation of hepatitis C was a discovery itself made possible by the isolation of hepatitis B in 1966 by Baruch Blumberg, working at the NIH. Blumberg won the Nobel Prize for Medicine but didn't get fabulously wealthy. Back in the good old days, people thought winning a Nobel was evidence of the highest achievement possible for human beings and was, therefore, its own adequate reward.

person, although the route of transmission is unknown in about 25 percent of people who get hepatitis C.

The CDC believes there are more than three million Americans with undiagnosed hepatitis C, some of whom will develop cirrhosis, liver failure, and cancer of the liver as a result of their chronic infection, but only after ten to thirty years of showing no symptoms while still spreading the virus. Many people with hepatitis C will live normal life spans and will never develop symptoms of the disease, making the calculus about who and when to treat more complicated. Deaths from hepatitis C became more common than deaths from HIV as the infected baby boomers aged and began to develop symptoms. Hepatitis C is problematic in a different way than HIV, because it is less likely to be symptomatic and less likely to be immediately life-threatening when it does become symptomatic, so many more people can have it, spread it, and never seek treatment, and it is more likely to spread unseen and undetected.

The people most likely to have undiagnosed hepatitis C are baby boomers born between 1947 and 1965. The CDC recommends that all members of this cohort be screened, but few are. The problem with hepatitis C may becoming worse, given the opiate overdose epidemic of 2013 to the present, as many more people are using injectable illicit drugs and may be spreading both HIV and hepatitis C, although we haven't yet seen evidence of that spread in the data we collect from the limited random screening we now do.

There have been treatments for hepatitis C since the mid-1990s, but the early treatments were moderately expensive, not very effective, and made you sick while you were taking them. In 2014, very effective treatments that are well tolerated became available, but they cost $84,000 a person at first. "Competition in the market" reduced the cost to "as low as" $63,000 a person. For people who know they have hepatitis C and who discovered it while they were healthy, the decision about taking the hepatitis

C medication is a challenging one. Some insurance companies don't cover the cost of the medication until the virus does permanent damage to your liver, because they know that many people with hepatitis C will never get sick. But few people who can afford $63,000 or $84,000 are willing to gamble, so almost everyone who screens positive and can possibly afford it gets treated. The profit margin for the drug manufacturers is huge, so it is in their interest to encourage every baby boomer to be screened because everyone who screens positive is a new customer. At the same time, treatment definitely saves lives. As with HIV, much of the drug purchase for hepatitis C medications is funded by Medicare and Medicaid, in part because many people who are using or have used injectable drugs qualify because of poverty or age. So hepatitis C treatment represents a huge success for biotech science, a lifesaving treatment, a reminder about the need for a health care system that would allow us to screen everyone at risk for hepatitis C, a source of tremendous profit for pharmaceutical companies, and a transfer of public resources into private pockets, all at the same time.

It's a morally ambiguous situation. On the one hand, we have a dangerous disease that is widespread in the population and that will sicken and kill many of the people who get it. On the other hand, drug companies and their stockholders make huge profits on the fears and misfortunes of many Americans, profits often funded by the American taxpayer.

To make our moral quandary a little more difficult, let's try another thought experiment. Would we be having this discussion at all if hepatitis C treatment were free? Even more, would we be having this discussion if everyone at risk had been screened in 1992, if everyone who was hepatitis C positive was identified and adopted behaviors to limit the spread of the disease?

One more note about hepatitis C that bears on the consequences of our failure to have a health care system in the U.S. I first saw how dangerous for-profit medicine is for democracy in 1999, when I was a practicing family doctor helping to create an occupational disease clinic. In order to push back against a local manufacturer that had caused a new occupational disease and against a hospital in cahoots with the manufacturer that had fired a brilliant researcher and colleague, I teamed up with the labor union movement and others to help build a new occupational health clinic. This new clinic was independent of any hospital and so could not easily be shut down—so it could, in the language of the time, serve the people. One colleague in this effort was a well-known local labor leader who had impeccable left-wing credentials. One day that labor leader mentioned he was on his way to Puerto Rico for a weekend of golf.

"That sounds pretty cool," I said. "Do you go often?"

"No," said the labor leader. "Some drug company is flying me down. They make a medicine to treat hepatitis C, and they want us to start testing all the members of the firemen's union."

"Test the firemen's union?" I asked, still pretty naive.

"Oh yeah," the labor leader said. "All emergency medical technicians in the state belong to the firemen's union. They often get needle-stick injuries. And they transport lots of drug addicts, so someone figured out they are more likely to get hepatitis C."

"I don't get it," I said. "Why is a drug company flying you to Puerto Rico to play golf because some EMTs have hepatitis C?"

"Pretty simple," said the labor leader, who couldn't believe just how naive I was. "They fly me to Puerto Rico to play golf. I get them in with the firemen's union so we get all EMTs tested. They find cases of hepatitis C. All those guys have insurance. The guys with hepatitis C get treated. The drug company makes out like a bandit. And everybody's happy."

In 1999, that was where we were. We weren't testing and treating people with a serious disease because the disease was dangerous and we had a cure. We were bribing a labor leader to get his members tested so people with something to sell could make a profit. If it happened we could reduce the incidence and prevalence of disease and create a public benefit at the same time, then that was all well and good, but the driving force was profit, not the common good. My labor leader friend had no idea about the risks and benefits of treatment, and he didn't understand anything about the science behind the decision to treat, which at the time was pretty weak. No, instead of a health care system driving decisions in the public interest, we had for-profit corporations driving decision-making. All my labor leader friend knew was that he was getting a free trip.

What does our approach to hepatitis C say about who we have become, about our public health science, which has been subverted in the name of profit, about our public priorities, which are directed toward private profit and not the public good, and about our democracy? Does health care serve the public interest today or has it become just a way to make the rich richer and the poor poorer, as democracy is reduced to the status of a rapidly fading dream?

Things have only gotten worse since 2000, when my labor leader friend played golf in Puerto Rico.

When I was at the Rhode Island Department of Health in 2011, I learned about the scandal entailing 17-hydroxyprogesterone, a hormone that has a number of effects in the female reproductive cycle and has long been used to prevent recurrent premature labor in women who miscarry. It was first identified in 1929, first reproduced from animal tissue in 1934, partially synthesized from plant-derived compounds in 1940, and then synthesized in 1971. It has been available commercially since 1935. By the late 1990s, 17-hydroxyprogesterone was almost as cheap as water—less than five dollars a dose. Then the drug company that produced 17-hydroxyprogesterone withdrew it from the marketplace, afraid of potential product liability litigation and because there wasn't an adequate profit margin to justify its continued production. But the chemical from which the drug was made was widely and cheaply available. Pharmacists could easily make it out of precursors themselves, patient by patient, so it was available in every drug store in the U.S. for five to ten dollars a dose. That setup worked well for everyone for more than ten years.

By 2003, a number of studies began to appear that found 17-hydroxyprogesterone to be both safe and effective in preventing recurrent premature labor. Recurrent premature labor is a condition that causes a certain subset of pregnant women to deliver their babies early, often before the babies' lungs have matured, so those babies have to spend weeks or months in a neonatal intensive care unit at enormous expense, and too many of those babies die. Obstetricians began making wide use of 17-hydroxyprogesterone to prevent premature labor, improving our infant mortality rate and reducing the cost of health care. Even better, 17-hydroxyprogesterone helped us reduce an inequality associated with race—as infant mortality among children born to African Americans in the U.S. is three to four times greater than infant mortality among children born to white women, and African American women (particularly adolescents) are at greater risk for premature labor. Even better yet, 17-hydroxyprogesterone helps us reduce the public cost of health care, because, by about 2000, half of the babies born in the U.S. were born to women on Medicaid, so much of the cost of prematurity was being borne by the public purse. That cost was reduced with the help of 17-hydroxyprogesterone.

Up to 2011, it was all good. As a nation, we were working hard to reduce adolescent pregnancy, and we were succeeding despite conservatives in Congress who were doing their damnedest to make access to contraception more difficult for teenagers. By about 2014, we had cut the adolescent pregnancy rate in the U.S. to half of what it had been in the mid-1990s, a result of great public health work and cultural change, which made it okay for teenagers to be less sexually active, watered down a taboo, got us talking publicly about sex so that teenagers were able to better balance the social and biological forces in their lives, and allowed us to make good contraception more widely available. Fewer adolescent pregnancies. Less premature labor. We were even starting to make progress on the huge, devastating disparity in infant mortality between African Americans, Latinos, and the rest of the population.

Then in 2011, the 17-hydroxyprogesterone situation changed. KV Pharmaceuticals got the FDA to license the production and distribution of 17-hydroxyprogesterone as an orphan drug, which gave KV an exclusive license to market the drug for seven years.[10] KV marketed it under the trade name Makena, and the price went up. Way up. From $5 a dose to $1,500 a dose—with half the cost to be borne by state Medicaid programs and thus by the public itself.

Those of us who practiced medicine had been noticing this kind of behavior among pharmaceutical companies for a number of years. Drugs proven to be effective, which we knew well and were out of license so they were available inexpensively as generics, would suddenly disappear and then reappear as a wildly more expensive drug with a trade name. Some generic drugs disappeared altogether, as venture capitalists bought and then closed the factories that made those drugs to eliminate the generics, leaving only a single, licensed—and much more expensive—version of the drug available. The manufacturers were too often given a license because of a meaningless and trivial chemical change or a new "drug delivery" system. The

---

10 An orphan drug is a drug that treats a supposedly rare condition, one affecting fewer than two hundred thousand people, that would not be profitable for pharmaceutical manufacturers to market and distribute under normal market conditions. The Orphan Drug Act of 1983 gives manufacturers special considerations when a drug is declared an orphan drug.

trade-marketed drug would be ten or forty or a hundred times as expensive as the old tried-and-true generic.

In the case of 17-hydroxyprogesterone, one government agency (the FDA) found itself facilitating the for-profit activity of a for-profit company that created huge public cost, which had to be borne by another public entity—Medicaid. It is not possible for me to know how and why FDA rules enabled this transition, whether some smart lawyers found a loophole that could be used for private profit or whether drug company lobbyists got enabling legislation passed and regulations written in such a way as to open those loopholes. My guess is that it was a little bit of both. In the case of 17-hydroxyprogesterone, there was a public outcry that was just loud enough to get the FDA to change its tune a little, but not a public outcry that was fierce enough to change the for-profit and manipulative activity of drug companies as a whole. The FDA notified health professionals and pharmacists that it would not sanction pharmacists who continued to compound 17-hydroxyprogesterone and supply it for five to ten dollars a dose. KV Pharmaceuticals "dropped" the price of Makena from $1,500 a dose to $690 a dose, but they sent their lawyers to threaten every compounder of 17-hydroxyprogesterone with lawsuits, so most pharmacists stopped compounding it and selling it affordably. Medicaid programs just anted up and paid the freight, figuring that the savings they realized from reduced premature labor was worth the cost, regardless of how illegitimate the process that increased that cost was. (One small bit of justice—KV went bankrupt about a year later, despite its attempted extortion. But then it came out of bankruptcy, was sold, and then sold off the "rights" to Makena. Which still costs $690 a dose.)

When we were in the middle of the 17-hydroxyprogesterone debacle in Rhode Island, a faculty member who ran the compounding laboratory at the University of Rhode Island School of Pharmacy was ready to make the drug for anyone who needed

it in the state. URI could have supplied all the 17-hydroxypro-
gesterone Rhode Island needed for a price that was so low it
was almost free. One public entity could have fixed the problem
another public entity had created and saved taxpayers half a
million dollars a year—money that was being paid as tribute to
KV for its manipulation of the orphan drug approval process.
But the state's lawyers said no. Too much liability risk. We were
prevented from serving the public interest by one set of laws and
lawyers, so we couldn't fix a problem created by another set of
laws and lawyers, both of which had exploited the democratic
process to protect private profit over the common good. Rhode
Island just handed over public money to a private enterprise
that was smarter than us—and had better lawyers.

It's not just drugs. Every part of the health care enterprise has
now been opened to exploitation by for-profit companies. About
thirty years ago, we noticed that information about patients was
not being shared effectively between doctors and hospitals. All
our notes were handwritten—and often illegible—so they couldn't
be easily shared. Colleagues in other industries—banking
and finance, materials transport, and even automobiles—had
evolved electronic information systems that allowed them
to track the activities of individuals and to maintain records
of those activities over time. There is a public interest in the
free and easy exchange of medical information. That exchange
sometimes gets us critical information that we need quickly
when someone is desperately ill but more often should allow us
to avoid waste and errors if the information is made available
in a form we can understand. We can learn what medications a
person takes so we don't order medications that interact. We can
see recent lab tests and X-rays, so we don't order the same thing
over and over and expose patients to discomfort and radiation
unnecessarily. A well-put-together medical information system
could, one might think, make us more efficient, by not requiring

each health care practice, institution, and professional to obtain the same basic demographic and billing information from patients again and again.

You might think putting together a health information system that serves the public ought to be pretty easy. It's like building a highway system. Everybody needs roads and highways. You build them once, you build them well, and then all you have to do is maintain them. To make building a good health information system that serves the public even easier, it turned out we already had such a system in the U.S. It is called VistA and is the system that was used in the Veterans Affairs hospitals nationwide. I've never used it myself, but I hear it works pretty well. It needs customization, but it's free and public and tested.

But we didn't use VistA, and we didn't design another national health information system that included all Americans and that all health care professionals could learn and use. Instead, we allowed the marketplace to try to create electronic medical records, and that market created a zillion different computer programs that don't talk to one another. Nobody bothered to make it a system, so what we got was chaos. We sank more than $19 billion of public money into this mess, and I don't want to guess at the amount of private money that had to be invested as well. We now have many different electronic medical records systems and spend billions of dollars trying to get them to talk to one another—and they don't talk to one another well. Every health professional has to spend weeks learning the particularities and peculiarities of any electronic medical record they use—which are changing all the time. Most of us spend more time in examination rooms looking at the computer than we do looking at and talking with the person we are there to see and try to help. Want to know what's worse? The information on the screen is usually meaningless! I usually can't look up a patient's record and figure out what I need to know with a keystroke or two. I have to sit there and bounce from screen to screen and hope I figure it out correctly, because most screens contain acres and acres of meaningless lingo, all dreamed up to satisfy some bureaucrat who never touched a patient and wouldn't know what drug does what, even if the pharmaceutical company that made said drug mugged that bureaucrat in a back alley.

What we see here, in the case of drug company and health information company profiteering at the public expense is the vortex of for-profit health care and the way the profit motive can exploit medical services to create profit in the first place and to undermine democracy at the end of the day. We've allowed profit to become a legitimate goal of health care. That profit drains the public pocketbook and diverts our spending from needed social services like education and housing to spending that isn't necessary or is necessary but has become astronomically priced—like the trademarked version of 17-hydroxyprogesterone. The money that comes out as profit is spent on lobbyists who jigger the regulatory system in a way that allows more profit. Our education system begins to fail, and our people don't develop the analytic skills they need to advocate effectively for themselves or to stop the wholesale thievery out of the public pocketbook by people with something to sell. The lawyers and the lobbyists become more brazen and more effective at stealing from the public pocketbook, using health care as their justification. Then the cycle repeats itself, resulting in more and more centralization of wealth and power. The rich get richer, the poor get poorer, and the democratic process becomes a shadow of what it was, could be, and should be.

It's not just health care, of course. This focus on private profit is repeated in many other arenas: in education, with charter schools; in law enforcement, with private prisons; and in the military, with private contractors doing the dirty work of foreign interventions and foreign wars. But health care has proven to be a particularly potent arena for the transfer of public funds to the private pockets, as evidenced by the ever-growing slice of the gross domestic product devoted to health care spending.

In this way, health care costs and profiteering have become major contributors to the weakening of democracy, a weakening that will continue unless we all begin to understand what is going on in front of our eyes—and revolt.

We could have it another way, of course. We could recognize that health exists to make democracy stronger, allowing people to participate actively and knowledgably in the political process. We could make health care not-for-profit and charge our institutions with defending the common good. We could use our public universities to make those orphan drugs and old vaccines and supply them to all Americans without cost— funded by the taxpayer and free to the individual. We could set prices for new drugs, allowing some return on investment but not ungodly profits, so that we get a fair return on the huge public investment we make every year in basic science research and in building the careers of researchers and other academics. Researchers and academics ought to work for the common good and not for themselves, out of the pride of serving the nation, our democracy, and all humanity. We could create a health care system that cares for all Americans, paid for out of tax dollars, rather than jury-rigging a market to sell services, one that creates a role for insurance companies and pharmaceutical companies and a thousand other shysters with something to sell, who quite literally suck the blood out of the democratic process.[11]

I'm no communist. I think the market seems to work to develop goods and services that people need and want, and it is

---

11 Even blood banks have become virtual private enterprises focused on profit. They take donated blood and sell it to hospitals and dialysis centers and freestanding surgical centers for hundreds of dollars a pint, and they pay their executives hundreds of thousands of dollars a year.

an efficient way of distributing those goods and services to all the people who might want them. The market is a great way to sell tomatoes, cars, and TV sets. But the market just doesn't work for health care. Market-driven health care has failed to improve the public's health and to affordably accomplish the limited successes it has. We provide lots of essential services publicly— education, police and fire protection, water and sewage, airports and roads—and they work pretty well. Not perfectly but pretty well. And they are governed by a public process that can work to fix problems when they occur, should the public choose to be engaged and demand change. Our occasional shortcomings with how we manage one or more of those services are often cited as evidence that government doesn't and can't work. But all those services actually do work and, even better, are available to all Americans. Note that no one ever complains that we have socialized fire protection or socialized police, or even socialized education. Keeping government out of health care in the name of avoiding socialized medicine has proven a silly exercise in futility.

If government doesn't work perfectly, then we need to fix the damn government by participating in elections and in governing, instead of abandoning the most powerful instrument we have to help us provide this essential service to all Americans. The market has failed to produce health. Let's own that fact, juice up our democracy, make government function again, and bring a functioning government to bear on health care, and let's get it right this time.

When Jonas Salk announced success of the polio vaccine trial in 1953, he was reporting on a huge undertaking that involved 20,000 physicians and public health officers, 64,000 school personnel, 220,000 volunteers, and over 1,800,000 schoolchildren—and the whole world celebrated. Salk was widely hailed as a hero, and countries around the world—the U.S., Canada, Sweden, Denmark, Norway, West Germany, the

Netherlands, Switzerland, and Belgium—immediately began polio immunization campaigns using Salk's vaccine.

It is estimated that the Salk vaccine was worth $7 billion, but Dr. Salk refused to patent it. His only interest was the betterment of humankind, not personal profit. When asked who owned the patent to it, Salk said, "There is no patent. Could you patent the sun?"

Our attempt to use the patent process to make health a commodity and to use the market to "distribute" health has been a miserable failure. If all this private enterprise were justified, both HIV and hepatitis C would have been eliminated by now, the rate of prematurity would be much reduced, the infant mortality rate would be less, we'd have thirty thousand fewer deaths a year from influenza, longer life spans, and we'd have an electronic medical records system that would let us get all Americans the prevention they need, enabling us to find people who are at risk for disease and early death and mitigate those risks—and probably do even more than that.

Big Bill Haywood famously said that when one man had a dollar he didn't work for, some other man worked for a dollar he didn't get. So when somebody's making more money off health care than they need at the public's expense, while the rising costs contribute to income inequality, then you and I are paying for healthy lives and a healthy democracy that we aren't getting.

It's time to dump our market approach to health care. We need a health care system that cares for all Americans, and we need that health care system now.

CHAPTER THREE

What Matters for Health

ROSETO, PENNSYLVANIA, CAME TO THE WORLD'S NOTICE IN THE YEARS 1935 TO 1985, because the people who lived there weren't having heart attacks and dying of heart disease in a period when heart disease was the most significant cause of premature death in the U.S.[1] Citizens of Roseto had a vastly lower incidence of heart disease than did people who lived in neighboring towns, the state of Pennsylvania, or the nation as a whole, despite the fact the people who lived in Roseto ate a diet that was no better than the places to which it was compared and didn't exercise more. Instead, Roseto had something more powerful: a connected and engaged community and family-focused population of people who lived together in one place and intended to keep doing that.

Roseto is a little town of 1,600 in the hills of northeast Pennsylvania that had been shaped by a culture of community cohesion and family solidarity. It was settled in 1882 by a group of Italian immigrants who all came from Roseto Val Forte, a town in the province of Foggia in southern Italy, and its culture was shaped by a dedicated and sophisticated parish priest named Father Pasquale de Nisco, who functioned as confessor, de facto mayor, community organizer, and moral authority for Roseto's people. Father de Nisco built Roseto into a place where

---

1   John G. Bruhn and Stewart Wolf, *The Power of Clan: The Influence of Human Relationships on Heart Disease* (New Brunswick, NJ: Transaction Publishers, 1993).

families stayed together and people took care of one another, where what mattered were relationships, not income or social prominence.

In 1961, a physician in a nearby town noticed that people in Roseto weren't dying of heart disease, and his chance comment to a colleague about that fact triggered a huge epidemiological investigation. Scientists came to see for themselves. They studied death certificates. They tested the water and tracked people's diets and physical activity. They got people to fill out questionnaires. And they found that the people of Roseto were only half as likely to die of the heart disease as were people in surrounding communities. What's more, those scientists found that the reduced risk of heart disease wasn't the result of genetics or diet or the mineral content of the local water or physician skill or the presence of obesity, diabetes, high blood pressure, or even infectious disease. The scientific evidence suggested that social cohesion—the impact that living in a close, connected community—was preventing heart disease. Just when small towns in the U.S. were falling apart, just when extended families were breaking apart, just when the nuclear family itself was beginning to disintegrate, Roseto suggested that family and community mattered for health, that family and community might help prevent heart disease.

This hypothesis was validated in the second half of the study, from 1965 to 1985, when the social cohesion of Roseto started to fall apart. As pressure from consumerism disrupted the social cohesion of Roseto, the rate of heart disease and heart disease death in Roseto rose to the same level as the surrounding communities and the nation as a whole.

Since the Roseto study, we've developed mountains of evidence that is more sophisticated statistically, and this evidence tells the same story over and over again. Social cohesion matters for health. Our healthiest places are those where people stick together enough to educate their children and protect the environment, where housing is safe and few people are home-less, where fewer people drink or smoke or do drugs. We can design whatever health care system we want. We can build hospitals or not. Train he..th professionals or not. Have copays or not. Use the market or not. But as we think about what works, we need to remember that we must build and strengthen communities if we are to be effective in improving the health of Americans, so building and strengthening communities needs to become the focus of our health care enterprise. It is just easier for Americans to be healthy if we live in communities where people know one another and can take care of their own.

The first intellectual problem that underlies the failure of our health care market to make the U.S. a healthier nation is that Americans don't share a clear understanding of what health is, so we don't know what we are trying to achieve by spending all this money—which gives everyone license to spend money on everything. The second intellectual problem underlying the failure of our health care market to make us healthier is a certain fuzziness about cause and effect in health and health care—confusion about what we can or should do to create healthier people and a healthier population. The third intellectual problem is that the measures we use to understand what we mean by the health of individuals and the health of the population don't accurately reflect what we mean by health at the end of the day.

Health is a broad but vague concept like Love or Justice. Health serves as a goal that can motivate the population to act, but health as an idea can just as easily be exploited and manipulated by people with something to sell. That's because every person defines health differently for himself or herself. Most of us think about health as one part the ability to function as a member of a family or community, one part freedom from pain, and one part the ability to live a long time, with each of us mixing the proportion of those concepts together in different ways. When we talk about public health, on the other hand, we are referring to two separate and distinct concepts. One concept is the commonsense perception of social or environmental conditions that impact the health of individuals. A crowded slum or a contaminated public water supply, for example, is said to be bad for the public's health. But public health also refers to a set of measurable overall characteristics of the population that allow us to compare different places. We measure and discuss life expectancy, for example, when we compare Japan to China, or infant mortality, when we compare New York to Utah, or when we compare the social condition and experience of African Americans and Latinos to Americans of European descent. Life expectancy, infant mortality, years of potential life lost, the likelihood that a particular disease or condition will develop in different proportions of the population of a place—which epidemiologists, who are really population health scientists, call the incidence and prevalence of that disease or condition—these are some of the measures we use to understand and think about how social organization and the environment impact the people who live in different places.[2]

In an earlier book, James Peters and I proposed a practical definition of individual health to guide public policy, and that's

---

2   It is worth noting that many important impacts of social organization cannot currently be measured, so they slip under our analytic and intellectual radar. We lack good measures of social trust at the community level, of community engagement or involvement, and of the happiness, comfort, and joy of people living in a place. The suicide rate and the incidence and prevalence of drug and alcohol addiction gives us some measure of the despair or unhappiness of individuals who live in a certain place, but we don't measure the success of those communities at helping community members build meaningful lives. Sometimes what we measure impacts what we do, even when what we measure isn't that important, so it is helpful to be mindful about what is not measured, so we don't forget to attend to it.

the definition I'll fall back on here.[3] Health, we argued, is the equal ability of individuals to function in family and community at any point in the life cycle and to actively participate in the democratic process. And public health is a set of measures that allows us to compare the environmental conditions and social organization of places. In that book, we didn't articulate the purpose of medical services or of what passes for a health care system in a community or a place. It is that purpose I hope to explicate here.

Definitions aside, it is important to understand what matters, which programs and processes help people achieve the goals that we measure when we talk and think about the health of individuals and places. Such an analysis helps us understand the extent to which our public spending on goods and services is effective at achieving the goals we intend to achieve. How good is what we buy with public money at improving health as we understand it? What can or should we buy to improve the health of the population, and what can or should we buy to improve that health most efficiently and effectively?

As previously noted, we now spend about $3 trillion a year on goods and services intended to improve health. Of that spending, 30 to 40 percent goes to hospitals and 20 percent to doctors—mostly to specialists. Drug purchases account for another 20 percent, and 20 percent is spent on things like equipment and supplies—for example, breathing machines and crutches and those cool little scooters people drive along the sides of streets that are so effectively advertised on TV.

But here's the hard news. Very little of what we buy matters much for health, or at least matters much when it comes to reducing infant mortality, increasing life expectancy, reducing years of potential life lost, or creating community, happiness,

---

3   Michael Fine and James W. Peters, *The Nature of Health: How America Lost, and Can Regain, a Basic Human Value* (Oxford: Radcliffe Publishing, 2007).

and joy—however difficult it is to measure or meaningfully discuss those goals. Vaccines and vaccinations matter for life expectancy. Medicines probably help people with diabetes, heart disease, high blood pressure, HIV, and hepatitis C live longer. Seeing the doctor right away when you are pregnant reduces the likelihood that you will lose your pregnancy, although about one-third of all pregnancies are not carried to term, even in 2017, despite all our fancy technologies. Having ambulances, doctors, and hospitals available when a natural disaster strikes probably reduces the loss of life and the extent of disability from injury, but natural disasters occur infrequently, so this impact on the population as a whole is hard to detect statistically.

But there is no clear evidence that any of the rest of it matters—the doctors, the hospitals, the breathing machines, and even the cool little scooters driving alongside streets—at least from a public health perspective (even though many of those services provide comfort and perhaps even a few extra years of life to individuals who become ill). We don't know if the number and location of hospital beds has any impact at all on the longevity or function of the population. But there is good evidence that too many hospital beds is associated with greatly increased cost and some adverse health impacts, because hospitals work hard to fill their empty beds, leading them to do too much to people who weren't really sick. On the other hand, there is some evidence that the number, location, and organization of maternity services do impact infant mortality, though they are not the strongest predictors of infant mortality by any means. Other factors—early prenatal care, nutrition, time off from work, and other social supports—have a much greater impact and cost a whole lot less.

The same is true of doctors. There is good evidence that the number and location of primary care doctors (family physicians, internists, and pediatricians) are associated with less infant mortality, longer life expectancy, fewer deaths from heart disease and cancer, and lower costs. But the number and location of other specialists are associated with shorter life expectancy and higher costs. Two-thirds of the doctors in the U.S. are specialists, which is one of the ways in which we are different from other countries—many of which have medical communities that are half to two-thirds generalist physicians.

But no one knows *how* generalists impact public health. Yes, having more primary care doctors means more people will be screened for preventable diseases—something primary care doctors do adequately but not brilliantly. Yes, primary care doctors provide more vaccinations, again adequately but not brilliantly, as they, in partnership with school nurses and legislation that requires vaccination for school, make sure more than 80 percent of American kids are adequately vaccinated. (A much smaller proportion of the adult population is adequately vaccinated, despite our having lots of primary care doctors for adults.)

Some of us think that the impact of primary care in the health care market we have now comes from protecting the public from the rest of the health care system. When you go to see your family doctor for a headache, she or he is likely to know your family and your personal situation and stresses. He or she will ask you about how you are sleeping and will check on your neck and back—which is where most headaches actually come from—and will figure out a way to treat your headache effectively in one visit. When you go to the emergency department for a headache, you'll see doctors who don't know you or your family and community, and they'll give you a CT scan and an MRI and perhaps a spinal tap because they're worried about all the terrible things they see commonly but occur rarely and are devastating causes of headaches, like brain tumors and aneurysms. You'll also generate a $5,000 to $10,000 bill and leave with instructions to get a neurology consultation, which may lead to more tests and procedures, most of which are likely unnecessary, and all of which carry a small statistical risk. Multiply that small statistical risk by all the people who go to the emergency room with a headache, and you get the increased risk of injury and death caused by the medical services marketplace. The *British Medical Journal* recently estimated that in the United States something like 250,000 deaths yearly result from medical errors and the overuse of medical services—and that doesn't include injuries.[4] The costs associated with all these unnecessary medical services are astronomical.

What primary care doctors do probably doesn't affirmatively improve the public health much. But primary care doctors are valuable because people who use primary care don't use the specialty and hospital care, which is dangerous when not necessary. Yet that specialty and hospital care consumes about 50 to 60 percent of our health care spending, or about $1.8 trillion a year. So having lots of primary care doctors matters a little for health, but mostly because they protect people from the rest of a health care market out of control.

Most of us think no more than 10 percent of public health outcomes are due to medical services—the services that consume $3 trillion a year.[5] The 10 percent estimate is a wild guess, widely believed but based on no real evidence. No one knows the real number, but I'd be surprised if medical services are even that effective, despite consuming 18 percent of the gross national product. Remember that public health outcomes are only indicators that we are able to measure to help us compare the social organization and environmental conditions in *different*

4   Martin A. Makary and Michael Daniel, "Medical Error—The Third Leading Cause of Death in the US," *The BMJ* 353, no. 2139 (May 3, 2016), available at https://www.bmj.com/content/353/bmj.i2139 (accessed April 30, 2018).

5   Steve A. Schroeder, MD, "We Can Do Better—Improving the Health of the American People," *New England Journal of Medicine* 357, no. 12 (September 20, 2007): 1221-28, available at https://www.nejm.org/doi/full/10.1056/NEJMsa073350 (accessed April 30, 2018).

places—life expectancy, infant mortality, and the like—and don't reflect our ability to function in community, our happiness, comfort, our joy, or our ability to participate in the democratic process, which is what most of us really mean by health.

If only 10 percent or less of public health outcomes are a function of medical care (which consumes $3 trillion a year), what produces the other 90 percent of the public's health? If medical care doesn't matter much for public health outcomes, what does matter? And what would happen if we spent our money on those things that matter, instead of what doesn't seem to matter much?

Sanitation matters. Clean water, the proper disposal of waste, and the safety of food matter a lot. We started to understand food and water safety in the mid-1800s with the work of Rudolf Virchow, John Snow, and others. They used epidemiology—the classic analytic tool of public health—to help track down patterns of infectious diseases like cholera and found the sources of that infection in contaminated water and food, which led us to create safe public water systems and develop standards for food safety, so, beginning in about 1900, we were able to prevent illness and death from many infectious diseases. Sanitation in health care itself matters. Basic hand hygiene and the use of sterile procedures in operating rooms and by people like dentists and acupuncturists, people giving shots, and even tattoo artists matters. Procedures that help secure the safety of the blood supply also matter, because a safe blood supply prevents medical services from doing affirmative harm, even when we can't prove they do measurable good.

Infection control by departments of health matters. Infectious diseases are naturally occurring phenomena that change and evolve over time and take advantage of the proximity of human beings to one another to spread. Outbreaks of infectious disease can be controlled by good public health practice: by identifying people who harbor diseases and treating or isolating them and their contracts. Good public health practice saves lives. New diseases like Ebola and Zika will emerge and threaten the population every few years, and a healthy society is one that is prepared to use good public health practice to contain, control, and prevent those diseases with new vaccines and environmental controls.

Sanitation and control of infectious disease, broadly defined, were put into practice in the years around and just after 1900 and had much to do with the doubling of the expected life span between 1900 and 2000. Everyone benefited when we put these measures in place. That's the good news. The bad news is that these measures now exist. With the exception of a (relatively) small additional investment in our public health infrastructure that would help us better combat infectious disease, more public or private spending on sanitation will not yield much more public health improvement as measured by life expectancy and infant mortality.

Safe and healthy housing and a clean environment matter. Our industrial history created a world in which people were crowded together and exposed to a variety of environmental poisons that wrecked our lungs and gave too many of us cancer. Crowded housing created the conditions in which many people were exposed to and contracted tuberculosis. Social compression—the effective isolation of lots of poor people and those with disabilities into places with few social services—gives way to violence and drug and alcohol use. The lead-based paints used in urban environments left a legacy of contaminated dust and soil that still sickens our children today. We can make some progress improving public health indicators like life expectancy, infant mortality, and health disparities by race by building new housing and by renovating and cleaning those old industrial sites. Investment in housing is money well spent.

Not smoking matters. Cigarette smoking and other tobacco use is the leading preventable cause of potential years of life lost in our population. We need to end it forever, and any money we spend doing that will be money well spent.

Drug and alcohol use matters. Drug overdose is the leading cause of death among people eighteen to sixty-four. Someone makes a profit—legally or illegally—every time anyone picks up a shot glass or takes a toke or does a hit. Drug and alcohol addiction is a complex social challenge. Only 10 percent of us are susceptible to addiction, which means the other 90 percent of us are able to enjoy some moderate use without a high risk of developing dependence. The challenge of our public policy is to allow some use and some profit but to work together to prevent the addiction that sometimes results from casual use and to treat the addiction—itself a disease—when it emerges in some of the individuals who consume. Prevention of widespread use and addiction is a critical public health priority, and treatment of people with a substance use disorder is and ought to be a central public health priority.

Food and nutrition matters a lot. We have created epidemics by allowing the mass marketing of meat that raises cholesterol and industrial food products and sugar-sweetened beverages that cause obesity, and then high blood pressure, heart disease, stroke, and diabetes, which itself leads to kidney failure, heart disease, and blindness. Much of the food sold in our supermarkets, bodegas, and fast-food restaurants is toxic, and that we allow it to be sold at all suggests there is a bankruptcy in our public process. Knowing that, we ought to stop subsidizing dangerous goop and start subsidizing and promoting fresh fruit and vegetables. Imagine a world in which apples and carrots are promoted the way Oreos and Cheetos and Coke are promoted now.

How might we approach stopping the epidemic of obesity and diabetes? First, we ought to tax the hell out of industrial food-like products that are mass marketed and that too many people eat too much of. Industrial food-like products include anything that comes wrapped in a flavor-sealed pouch, anything sold in a fast-food joint, and anything artificially sweetened. That's potato chips and most breakfast cereal, nachos, Lunchables, McDonald's burgers, and french fries in all their incarnations—basically anything that isn't fresh fruits and vegetables, including soda and most fruit juices. All that goop is directly harmful, because industrial food science is very good at making it taste so good that we keep coming back for more. They've proven, though billions of dollars of profits, that we can't eat just one. So we need to tax the goop and use the tax dollars to build local agriculture, public transportation, and community centers. And we need to tax, not subsidize, the production or corn, wheat, and sugar to cut off the problem at its source, because none of these crops are needed now to maintain the diet of a healthy population.

Public transportation and community institutions matter. Public transportation has two important impacts. First, you have to walk a little bit to and from the bus or the train, and that walking is good for you. Second, you see other people on the bus and the train, and that human contact is also good for you. Americans forget that not so many years ago, we had community centers—YMCAs and Boys and Girls Clubs. We had places to go and hang out after work or after school, places with a gym and a pool, in pretty much every community. Kids would have a place to go and play ball after school and on weekends, and adults had places to spend time together, exercising or learning in adult education centers. Yes, some community centers and many Ys still exist, but their social role has been supplanted by for-profit gyms and fitness centers. Many of those allow people who are motivated to stay fit, which is a good thing, but the for-profit nature of the enterprise means we have segregated our world into those who can afford the fancy gyms and those who can't. It would be better for us to build community centers for everyone, build exercise into our daily life, and use our resources to create other publicly funded places for us to be together—museums, concert spaces, theaters, and public parks—than to allow ourselves to be so easily divided by income and culture.

Can I prove that taxing industrialized food products and using the money to subsidize local agriculture, build better public transportation, and making sure there is one community center for every community will reduce diabetes and save lives? Of course I can't. No well-standardized, double-blind crossover trial has ever been done to prove that, and none ever will be. Such a trial is too complex and too expensive. But no well-standardized, double-blind crossover trial has ever been done on our market-driven industrial food system either. In fact, our demand for evidence-based decision-making in all our public processes is helping to drive our market culture, because evidence is controlled by market actors who can afford to obtain it and know how to ask research questions that are inherently biased. One of the challenges in our public life is the challenge of using a certain amount of suggestive evidence mixed with a certain amount of common sense to make good decisions that benefit all of us. And we also have to use a certain amount of moral courage to not let ourselves be so easily picked apart by people with something to sell.

Physical activity matters. It's the best defense against obesity, diabetes, high blood pressure, heart disease, and stroke. But we've engineered physical activity out of our lives. It is relatively easy to build physical activity into our cities and towns, using bike paths and well-engineered walking routes through pedestrian malls closed to car traffic, and easier still to create a social consensus exercise around using the stairs instead of elevators and having kids walk to school together, by having adults walk with them as a group in what's called a walking school bus—but those things won't happen unless we put our mind to them. Let's close all city centers to private cars during normal working hours; let's find ways to provide incentives for people who are not disabled to use the stairs rather than elevators.

Education matters—though indirectly. People who are more educated live longer, have less infant mortality, and make more money. Higher-income people live longer and have less infant mortality (although it's interesting to note that poor people are nicer to one another—or at least contribute a higher proportion of their salaries to charity). There's nothing magic about education from a biological perspective. There is no change in the body or the immune system that results from taking three or five college courses. Educated people have just learned to make healthier choices. They chose healthy social connections. They learn why not to smoke and drink, and some of them even learn to avoid doctors and hospitals unless it is absolutely necessary. We don't know with certainty that investment in education will create a healthier population, because again, no one has ever done the well-designed, double-blind crossover trial to prove that education creates better public health outcomes. But the association between education and public health outcomes is so strong that an investment in public education seems wise, and the importance of an educated population for a meaningful democracy is more vital than much of our spending on medical care.

Race matters for health but, again, indirectly. There are mountains of evidence showing African Americans and Latinos have poorer health outcomes than white Americans. Race as we measure it is a proxy measurement for racism, which, to paraphrase Ezra Pound, might be called a stupid suburban prejudice, but it's a prejudice that has bedeviled the lives of too many Americans in ways too numerous to count. Race influences health through a number of mechanisms: through stress, poverty, education, and reduced access to medical care. It's interesting that even though too much access to medical care has some association with adverse health outcomes in the population as a whole, improved access to primary care has been shown to reduce health disparities among the women and children of the African American population. But primary care isn't anywhere near powerful enough to outweigh the deleterious effect of racism on the health of individuals and has almost no effect on the health of African American men, who often bear the brunt of the public expressions of institutional racism and are too often hassled by police and selectively imprisoned, resulting in an epidemic of incarceration among black men, itself independently associated with poor health outcomes.

The challenge in our thinking about race and racism as markers for public health outcomes, however, is the problem of how to change the impact of race. There is no drug to treat the stupidity of people who perpetuate racist beliefs and practices. And though social and economic reparations can help address the damage a history of racism has wreaked on generations of American families, there is no medical treatment to repair that damage per se, although we use health care to treat some of the biologic and social impacts of the harm racism has caused—more high blood pressure, diabetes, and stroke, more premature delivery and infant mortality, and many more victims of violence. And there is a mountain of evidence showing that the victims of racism are not treated equally by our dysfunctional health care market, even with improved access to health insurance. We need to use our regulatory agencies to ensure equal treatment. We need to make primary care and specialty care (primary care specifically) available to every person who has to live in a racist society and might be harmed by it, but health care itself won't fix racism. Our society as a whole has to do that by owning our past, confronting the bias that exists in every one of us, and then changing our racist beliefs, practices, and institutions.

Some of our public health spending needs to be devoted to doing the kind of analysis that makes sure people are treated equally by our health care institutions and professionals. We need to keep a focus on the elimination of health disparities associated with race as part of every decision we make about public spending on health and medical services. Income inequality is the intellectual bugaboo of our thinking about what matters for health. Lots of studies show that there is an association between income inequality and poor public health outcomes, although public health scientists are far from a consensus on this indicator and its association with health. Some have suggested a biologic mechanism by which income inequality might create poor outcomes: people are more stressed where there is social distance between people of different income levels, and stressed people fire up their adrenergic nervous system (the fight-or-flight reaction). A chronically fired-up fight-or-flight nervous, circulatory, and hormonal system causes hardening of the arteries, high blood pressure, and stroke. Places where there is a big divide between rich and poor have more social unrest, the argument goes, and that causes more stress.

In the U.S., we think more about poverty than we do about income inequality. Poor people don't have access to fresh fruit and vegetables, so they rely on high-calorie, high-salt, and industrial food products for their nutrition, and consuming that kind of food causes diabetes, heart disease, and stroke. Illness is also associated with more poverty. Poor people sometimes live in city neighborhoods near factories and mills or where factories and mills used to be, so they are exposed to old industrial pollutants and are much more likely to be lead poisoned. So yes, there is a real association between poverty, income inequality, and public health outcomes.

We have no have evidence and aren't likely to get evidence that reducing income inequality will improve public health outcomes. A number of previously discussed social factors associated with income inequality and poverty—education, housing, environment, food nutrition, physical activity, freedom from tobacco use, and effective prevention and treatment of drug and alcohol use and addiction—are predictors of poor health outcomes, so our public spending on health ought to target these factors. Reducing income inequality is a social good in its own right, because more equality creates more social peace, and social peace creates the conditions under which democracy is most vibrant, and vibrant democracy prevents social instability, and social instability, when it occurs, is bad for everyone's health. Peace is better than war. Justice is better than injustice. I don't need to make reference to better public health outcomes to make those claims, and I keep hoping that my friends and colleagues who want to use income inequality to justify the need for social justice and democracy will realize that social justice and democracy are values that deserve our support in and of themselves.

As the discussion about Roseto, Pennsylvania, showed, social coherence—the extent to which people in a place get along and are willing to spend time together and work together to build a meaningful common life—appears to matter a lot for health, but like education, racism, and income inequality, social coherence is an influencer, an intellectually slippery notion when viewed in the context of health. There aren't clear measures of social coherence that everyone understands and agrees on the way we understand and agree on infant mortality or life expectancy. The measures we try to use, measures like the number of voluntary associations per person or the extent to which we trust one another as measured by surveys, are all associated with better classic public health outcomes. Those measures tell us that places that have more social trust are associated with longer life expectancy, less infant mortality, and so on.

Part of the intellectual problem with the associations between social coherence and health is a lack of scientific consensus about the validity of the measures of social coherence, which are all self-defined. The definition of a voluntary association, for example, differs from person to person, and the meaning or intensity of the extent to which we trust someone is pretty subjective, try as we may to design survey instruments that are consistent and establish internal validity. Mortality is hard and measurable—everyone can count the years you live and we all count years in the same way. But there is also the sense that social coherence *is* health, which is why the argument that social coherence matters for health appears circular. If social coherence is a necessary condition for health, it is hard to say a necessary condition matters in the same way as we say a material condition matters. If we provide better sanitation and better food, we'll get a healthier population. But we can't provide more social coherence in the same way. When we create a healthier population, we get more social coherence. When there is more social coherence, when we are getting along and spending more time together, the population's health improves. When the population's health suffers illness, when there is an epidemic, a natural disaster, or an increase in substance abuse and drug overdose death, our ability to be together safely and comfortably is diminished, and social coherence suffers—the world becomes every man or woman for him or herself. When our social coherence is fraying, we feel unsafe but not necessarily unwell. Cause and effect in regard to health and community is hard to establish, because health and community overlap, as necessary conditions for one another.

Still, from a public health perspective, if you gave me a choice between building a hospital or a library or school, I'd choose the library or school every time, at least until the moment there was an outbreak of a disease that hospitals help treat. And because libraries are much cheaper than hospitals, you can build ten or twenty libraries for the cost of one new hospital building and serve hundreds more people every day.

That's the tension that exists when we think about public spending, health, and medical care. Spending on medical care helps address our fear of the unknown, though it isn't effective at all in improving the public's health. Spending on social programs (sometimes) helps make a more vibrant society if that spending is thoughtful and effective, and a vibrant society is more likely to make us healthier than will spending on medical care, particularly in our culture, where spending on medical care is more about someone else's profit than it is about our common life.

The way to improve the health of the population is to maintain sanitation and improve nutrition, housing, and the design of the built environment. Better education, a focus on addressing the impacts of a history of racism, and a concerted effort to eliminate cigarette smoking, cleaning the environment and keeping it clean, and the prevention and treatment of drug and alcohol addiction will make individuals and the public healthier. A health care system that can bring prevention to all Americans equally and that protects us from the overzealousness of some purveyors of medical care can make us healthier yet. Medical care provides treatment for and comfort to the sick. Sometimes. When it isn't killing the well. Medical care isn't health and it isn't a health care system.

Peace matters. It's impossible to be healthy when people are killing one another. If we have learned nothing from seeing the devastation caused by war in Syria, Liberia, or Gaza, we should at least learn that. Looking at war-torn places should help us value the democracy we have, which, however imperfect, allows us to maintain a social fabric that doesn't rely on violence to process our disagreements.

And democracy itself matters—perhaps even matters most. Democracy creates the social conditions that allow us to be at peace, at least domestically. Democracy channels our conflicts with one another into a forum that allows those conflicts to be resolved without violence, at least most of the time, so we are free to have relationships with one another. That we haven't been able to translate our relative domestic tranquility into an ability to avoid conflict internationally is a central failure of our democracy and our culture. Peace allows us to produce food and shelter and to create communities in which relationships can be sustained over time. Communities build housing and public transportation and protect the environment. We create health out of our relationships with one another, and then the health of the population circles back and makes democracy more robust. A health care system exists in that matrix of conditions and influencers to promote our ability to be in relationship with one another, so an effective health care system is one that focuses on the common good. Of all the material conditions and influencers that impact health, democracy matters most.

But the wealth extraction system that passes for health care in the U.S. is helping to destroy that democracy.

So maybe it's time to revolt.

CHAPTER FOUR

So What's Up with Obamacare?
Did It Matter?

TWENTY-THREE OR TWENTY-FOUR MILLION PEOPLE GOT HEALTH INSURANCE AS A result of the Affordable Care Act of 2010. About eleven million more signed up for Medicaid. About ten million people got subsidized insurance by buying insurance through the new health insurance exchanges, also called, unsurprisingly, health insurance marketplaces, and about 2.6 million young adults got to stay on their parents' insurance. The bad news, if you think health insurance is the Holy Grail, is that there are still about thirty million Americans who remain uninsured and more than ten million undocumented immigrants who have no chance of ever getting subsidized health insurance.

The other bad news is what all this cost. We spent a whole lot of money—$5-6 billion—just to build the health insurance exchanges, which allow only 6 percent of the U.S. population to buy insurance. The whole process increased the overhead cost of government and private insurance by $36 billion a year, or by about $1,873 per person newly insured—costs over and above the cost of the medical services we already provided.[1] That means we could have provided primary care for the rest of

---

1   David Himmelstein and Steffie Woolhandler, "The Post-Launch Problem: The Affordable Care Act's Persistently High Administrative Costs," *Health Affairs* blog, May 27, 2015, available at https://www.healthaffairs.org/do/10.1377/hblog20150527.047928/full/ (accessed April 15, 2018).

the nation's uninsured people for the same money we spend on the new administrative cost associated with the Affordable Care Act. Or, put another way, that means we chose to give money to insurance companies and government bureaucracy instead of providing direct service to those who need it most. And we spend a whole lot of public money altogether—something like $120 billion a year—which you'd think is a good thing, if you believe that insuring more people is worth the money. But it might not be that good, once you understand that a third to a half of every public dollar we spend on health care in the U.S. is unnecessary or wasted spending.

The 2008 election was an important opportunity to build a national consensus in favor of health care reform, and that national consensus was important in electing President Obama. But it wasn't clear enough or long-lasting enough to help us create a meaningful reform at the end of the day.

I was in Washington in March 2009 working at a primary care think tank and got to participate in some of the discussion at the stakeholder level, as policy makers tried to hammer out what health care reform should look like. I got to see the policy process at work and participate a little bit. Truth be told, the policy had been worked out long before the Obama campaign even got under way. All the drama of 2009 and 2010 was about figuring out what was politically possible on our way to enacting the predetermined reforms—the drama of negotiating around large stakeholders, who had enough money and who had assembled enough political power to deflect any changes that would impact their self-interest.

People hated health insurance companies and their arrogance. People wanted insurance that was affordable and reliable—that didn't promise to cover you and then dropped you when you were sick—and they wanted insurance that everyone could buy, because most people live in fear of not being able to afford health care should they get really sick. People also want hospitals and doctors to be there when they are sick, but most people don't perceive there is a problem with doctors and hospitals. The problems people were hearing about in 2008, 2009, and 2010 were problems with health insurance. Most people who thought about policy wanted a public option—a public insurance company that could compete with the private insurers that many perceived as corrupt and imperious. And many people on the left thought that we should do something about pharmaceutical companies and the way they were jacking up prices, though few of us had any clear idea what it was we should do.

Obamacare was health insurance reform. The Affordable Care Act requires all Americans to have health insurance of a certain type or face tax penalties and requires health insurance companies to sell people health insurance without regard to their existing health conditions. The Affordable Care Act also limits the difference in pricing of insurance products for people of different ages or genders, makes health insurance available to more people, and makes health insurance more affordable for lower-income people by subsidizing their purchase of insurance. But the act didn't make health insurance affordable over the long term, and it didn't require health insurance companies to offer the kind of health insurance people are required to buy.

The act changed health insurance to allow people younger than twenty-six to stay on their parents' insurance policy—a great advantage at a time when many young people did not have jobs that offer them health insurance. But we didn't change the critical underlying economic problem that created the need to allow those people under twenty-six to remain on their parents' health insurance policies in the first place—the fact that our economy has handicapped a generation of young people so they don't have enough income to buy health insurance for themselves. We didn't get a public option, which would have been a publicly owned insurance company that could compete with private insurers and was thought by some to be a useful way to keep insurance companies honest, because insurance companies used their lobbying power to stop the public option. And we didn't get bulk purchasing of pharmaceuticals and devices—a way to use the market power of the government to keep prices down—because Big Pharma used their lobbying power to outlaw bulk purchasing.

And we didn't build a health care system that provides the same set of services for all Americans regardless of race, culture, income, language, or geography.

If legislation is like making sausage, the Affordable Care Act of 2010 was an exercise in how to slice and dice anything and everything in sight and call what comes out the best sausage ever made, regardless of what went into making it. Politics is the art of the possible, and in 2010, truth be told, very little was possible in a democracy that had already allowed considerable income inequality and had already created a class of rich businesspeople with exceptional access to legislators and the legislative process.

If we are to understand why reforming health insurance didn't bring us health care that was effective and affordable, it is worth taking a moment to understand a little more about health insurance—about how it works, what it does, and how it is different from health care, about the business model of health insurance, and a little about what health insurance costs and why it is so expensive.

Health insurance is a business that promises to pay for medical care costs of individuals with money it collects regularly from or for individuals, pooling small regular payments from many people so that it can make large occasional payments for a few people. Health insurers make a profit by predicting the annual average health care cost, taking into account the large occasional costs of a few, and adding the costs of calculation and prediction, the cost of marketing the health insurers' offering, and profit, and by making sure that what the insurer charges is more than what the insurer has agreed to pay out. Insurers do better when they insure more people, because they have a larger incoming pool to balance the large occasional payout to individuals. They can also do better by writing carefully designed contracts that limit what they agree to pay for (though few of their customers understand those limits before agreeing to insurance contracts), by entering into agreements that limit what the insurer will pay for with doctors and hospitals, by making sure insurers only take customers who aren't likely to get sick, and by not continuing to make contracts with people who are sick and creating more expense.

The insurance industry is a place where all kinds of combinations, conspiracies, unholy alliances, and monopolistic behavior comes into play as market actors try to create and exert market power and leverage so that they can profit. Doctors and hospitals enter into contracts with insurers because insurers can send them paying customers, even though doctors and hospitals have to limit their charges and accept lower fees when they contract with insurers. Employers and other organizations that buy insurance for large numbers of people can get insurers to give up their right to refuse to insure individuals if those individuals have a preexisting conditions or should they get sick. Insurers are willing to give up that right in order to get a large number of customers at once, which creates predictable cash flow for insurers and helps them cover their overhead costs and secures their profit. Doctors and hospitals that join together to form larger organizations of health care providers in a market can force insurers to pay them better by threatening not to contract with them, because, at the end of the day, insurers need those doctors and hospitals to care for the people insurers insure, otherwise the products insurers offer become meaningless.

The real world of the health care and health insurance market in the U.S. is a dog-eat-dog world of promises made and broken, of organizations trying to create market power and use that market power to enrich themselves, of alliances, treaties, combinations, pacts, agreements, and betrayals, of shifting loyalties and the continuous hunt for leverage in pursuit of income and profit. With precious few exceptions, every actor in the health care marketplace is a private functionary pursuing private profit.

With precious few exceptions, no health care market actor has a public portfolio. No one voted this market in, per se, and no one has charged this market with the protection or promotion of the public's health. If and when some service that protects the public's health is made available by the market, the public health value is an accident. The market values and prices of services are based on demand and what the traffic will bear. In order to distribute services like vaccines that protect the public's health, the government has to enter the marketplace and use a public relations strategy—a form of public begging—to stimulate demand, and then has to beg hospitals and clinics and pharmacies to provide the service (which is exactly what we do for flu vaccine in flu season). The government turns out to have a weak mandate and few resources to protect the public's health. It has to either pay providers for offering and administering the service or has to create a regulation that requires the service as a precondition for access to another government provided benefit. But the government can't direct anyone to do anything in the service of the public's health, absent a natural disaster or a true public health emergency. Which means everyone concerned with health services—doctors, nurses, hospitals, nursing homes, insurance companies, pharmaceutical companies, device manufacturers—does exactly what they want to do and only what they want to do.

CMS, the government agency that runs Medicare and oversees Medicaid—the largest actor in the health care marketplace, government or otherwise—functions as a health insurer and not like a public health agency focused on health. It buys medical goods and services in the marketplace and uses pooled funds collected by the government, and while it doesn't make a profit, it is under lots of pressure from Congress, which acts as a group of shareholders, to drive down costs by negotiating with doctors, hospitals, and other service providers. That negotiation is very complex and involves Congress, lobbyists, and large national organizations, and because our public process is porous and open to influence by trade groups and lobbyists with money to spend, much of the negotiation is influenced by people with something to sell instead of being focused on the public interest. Medicare doesn't think out what services everyone needs and make sure everyone gets those services. It just decides what services it will pay for and lets doctors and hospitals decide whether to offer those services at the price Medicare will pay. The biggest and most powerful health care organizations use their lobbying power to make sure their services get paid best. The rich get richer and the poor get poorer, and that's all she wrote.

Health insurance was not originally created to fund predictable daily expenses of routine care. The health insurance market was poorly regulated early in its existence and moved into the "regular care" arena over time, because health insurance companies were able to garner considerable capital and market power and saw a vacuum in the market that would let them expand their market power even further. We use car insurance to protect us against the expense of car accidents but don't insure ourselves for the cost of oil changes and tune-ups. We have a social security, unemployment insurance, and a welfare system to protect ourselves from the personal risk of downturns in the economy and the hardships created by illness and aging and personal life chaos, but we don't insure ourselves for the cost of our groceries. The entrance of health insurance into the world of routine care might be thought of as something of a curiosity, except that entrance profoundly distorted the health care delivery system and allowed private corporations to usurp some of the traditional role of government, which is to provide necessary services to all Americans equally.

A good part of what the Affordable Care Act didn't do, however, was address itself to the delivery of health care services, but it is the character and availability of health services that makes health care more or less affordable and more or less effective at the end of the day. If there were a community health center open from 8:00 a.m. to 8:00 p.m. that would see you without a long wait, you'd use that when you were sick. But if your only choice is to call 911 and take an ambulance to a hospital emergency room, then that's what you'll do, even though that approach is ten times more expensive. When you're sick, you don't think much about health policy or even a whole lot about what things cost. There was and is no political consensus whatsoever about what the delivery of health care services should look like or about whether government has a role in structuring the delivery of those services. That's why the bulk of the Affordable Care Act didn't address service delivery, and that failure also explains why the Affordable Care Act has not made health care affordable or effective.

But the insurance market distorts the delivery system, and health care reform worsened that distortion. That distortion occurs because market power and not public health value rewards specific health care services and causes more of those services to be available. Public health and policy data show convincingly that we *need* relatively few hospitals and specialists and relatively many primary care clinicians, for example. But what we *have* is lots of hospitals and specialists and relatively few primary care clinicians. We *need* relatively few cardiologists and gastroenterologists but lots of addiction medicine specialists, psychiatrists, and other mental health workers, but we *have* lots of cardiologists and gastroenterologists and few addiction medicine specialists and psychiatrists—and most psychiatrists no longer accept insurance or Medicare at all! The Affordable Care Act, by failing to address itself to the public health value of medical services first or to create a medical services delivery system that focused on the public's health, failed to address the driver of health care cost in the U.S. and failed to create a way to improve the public's health at the end of the day. Health insurance in the U.S. is what's causing some of our problems, and the Affordable Care Act, by construing health insurance as the solution to those problems, made many of those problems worse.

Look at how we pay for primary care. Health insurance companies collect and distribute money. They make calculations so that their funds flow is adequate, they write contracts, and they market their products. Primary care clinicians care for between 1,500 and 2,000 patients; they are (or should be) available to their patients twenty-four hours a day, seven days a week. Primary care clinicians do their patients' physician examinations and see those patients when they are sick. Primary care clinicians fill out forms for work and forms for school and forms for life insurance companies. They help their patient decide when they need to see a specialist, who to see, and they tell the specialists about the patient's problem. Then they help the patient understand and make sense of the specialist's advice, coordinating the array of medical services available in a marketplace that exists only to sell services and not to actually help individuals make the best choices.

There is an avalanche of evidence showing that the number, location, and organization of primary care clinicians improves the public's health and helps control health care cost. The countries with the best primary care systems are those with the best health outcomes. The states with the greatest number of primary care physicians per hundred thousand people are the states with the lowest infant mortality rate, highest life expectancy, and lowest health care costs. If the health care market was working correctly to improve the public's health, we would be finding ways to improve the numbers of primary care clinicians and to make sure every American had a primary care clinician to work with. In most countries with high-performing health care systems, 50 percent or more of all physicians are primary care physicians and 50 percent are specialists. In the U.S. about 30 percent of all physicians are primary care and 70 percent of specialists, a ratio that hasn't changed in thirty years. That ratio would be considerably worse if the federal government, working through HRSA, hadn't intervened fifty years ago to create the community health center movement with programs that train more primary care clinicians and send them around the country, focusing on underserved areas.

The per-person per-year cost of health insurance is about $11,000. Of that, 10 to 20 percent—or $1,000-2,000 per person per year—stays with the insurance company, and the rest goes out, spent on health care costs of individuals. Between 3 and 4 percent—$400-500 per person per year—goes to primary care clinicians, and out of that income the primary care clinician has to pay staff and overhead before taking anything for him or herself. In order to get paid, primary care physicians and practices have to send a bill each time a patient walks through the door. They don't get paid a penny until that bill is sent. Most primary care physicians have to bill thirty to forty different health insurers, each with its own set of rules, so 20 to 40 percent of what primary care physicians earn is devoted to paying for the billing process itself. But the cost of primary care is an entirely predictable expense. Like the cost of groceries or routine care repairs, it is small enough that most people could actually afford it themselves. We could fix most of what ails health care in America if we just started paying primary care physicians and practices a certain amount of money per person per month and spread these physicians across the nation, so that there was a primary care practice or community health center in every neighborhood and community—unfortunately, reforming the health insurance industry did not give us the opportunity to do that.

Obamacare didn't change the balance of power in the health care market one bit. Insurance companies did better because Obamacare gave them twenty million new publicly funded customers. Pharmaceutical companies did better because they got twenty million new potential customers, and we agreed up front not to use the bulk purchasing power of the government to reduce drug prices. Hospitals did better because more of their patients are insured. So insurance companies, pharmaceutical companies, and hospitals became more powerful and more able to block any fundamental changes to the health care market.

But Obamacare brought primary care doctors a host of new requirements and responsibilities, and there has been none of the growth in the primary care sector we so desperately need. Primary care practices were already too busy, so having more patients didn't help. The tiny increases in payment primary care practices got in the reform were temporary and were accompanied by a whole new set of regulations and requirements that were expensive and difficult to address. Hospitals and community health centers did fine because the act reduced the number of uninsured people they care for.

Let me tell you about a thought experiment I did with colleagues at the Robert Graham Center in 2009. We modeled the costs and benefits of expanding access to insurance and compared that to the costs and benefits of providing primary care to all Americans in every community, applying the model developed by community health centers in the U.S. We predicted that expanding insurance alone to all Americans would cost $119 billion a year in new spending, in 2009. We also predicted that a health care system that provided primary care *and* health insurance to all Americans would generate between $59 billion and $371 billion a year in *savings*, not new costs, because deploying primary care keeps most of the population from overusing medical services. Our calculations suggested that providing primary care to all Americans would reduce infant mortality by 13 percent, which should save 31,625 lives. Life expectancy would increase by one full year for all Americans, heart disease mortality would decrease by 16 percent, which would save 102,000 lives and would reduce stroke mortality by 5 percent, which saves 6,000 lives. We presented this data on March 23, 2009, in the shadow of the Capitol—and the government policy makers who came to listen yawned. No one believed our numbers. *I* didn't completely believe the numbers because they were too good, even though the assumptions, though not perfect, were the best assumptions available at the time.

And then a few years later, when I was working at the Rhode Island Department of Health, which works closely with the CDC, I had occasion to review the CDC's Million Hearts Campaign. The CDC projected that if we could identify and control blood pressure in all Americans with high blood pressure, if we could identify all Americans with high cholesterol and reduce cholesterol, and if we could get daily aspirin to all Americans with known heart disease, we'd save two hundred thousand lives a year. Universal primary care—building a health care system instead of health insurance reform—does exactly those things and a whole lot more. The CDC's projection looked exactly like our projection—but suggested even more benefit. Writing this today, not having looked back at our projections for seven years, I went online to see what the Affordable Care Act—providing health insurance to many Americans but not all (we still leave out about thirty-three million people)—actually costs: $110–120 billion a year, depending on whether the sources are lovers or haters.[2] We underestimated both

---

2   Kerry Close, "Here's How Many Billions Obama Care Will Cost in 2016," *Money*, March 24, 2016, available at http://time.com/money/4271224/obamacare-chhost-taxpayers-2016/ (accessed April 15, 2018).

the cost of health insurance and the likely benefit of providing primary care to all Americans—of building a health care system to replace a failed marketplace—but our estimates were pretty close in both of those arenas. Now, looking backward, it is reasonable to think our estimates of the cost *savings* that might accrue from providing primary care to all Americans were pretty accurate as well.

No one should care about our ability to make estimates. But everyone should care about the missed opportunity to create a meaningful health care reform in 2010, a reform that should have improved public health outcomes, reduced income inequality, lowered health care costs, and strengthened, instead of weakened, our democracy.

No one yet knows whether the Affordable Care Act will have a net benefit from the perspective of the public's health. I'm betting there will be some very small, positive short- and medium-range net public health outcomes, which will come from providing preventive services to more people, but that those benefits will turn out to be incredibly costly.

I'm also betting that the long-term net public health benefit will be negative. We have seen income inequality continue to worsen in the U.S. in the period 2011 to 2015, the period when the Affordable Care Act was implemented. That's because the Affordable Care Act, in restructuring the health insurance marketplace, allowed already-rich insurance companies, pharmaceutical companies, hospital executives, and others to get richer, while health insurance premiums continued to climb faster than ever. Those increased expenditures took money out of the pockets of poor and working people despite the subsidies. The net financial effect of the Affordable Care Act is to transfer public funds away from public purposes and into the pockets of executives and stockholders of insurance companies, for-profit hospitals, and specialists.

The long-term net effect of the Affordable Care Act will probably be adverse. We will have improved or protected the health of some individuals but in a very expensive way, with the unintended consequence of widening the gap between rich and poor, creating a net negative public health consequence, and negatively impacting the democratic process, which is what our health care spending should be strengthening, not weakening.[3]

That said, Obamacare matters because we proved to ourselves that we actually can do health care reform, however imperfectly, when we as a people set our minds to it. Abba Eban famously said that Americans usually figure out the right answer after we've tried all the other ones. Let's call Obamacare one of the other answers, one we tried that failed to achieve what we needed to achieve, a way station on the road to building a health care system for everyone that makes democracy stronger, a health care system that is personal, affordable, rational, and just.

But perhaps we learned something more in 2009 and 2010. Perhaps our failure to effect meaningful reform helped us to understand that health insurance isn't health. Perhaps we also have started to understand that health care itself is unlikely to

---

3   Indeed, it appears that income inequality and wealth inequality have both increased between 2009 and 2015. Real income in the upper 1 percent increased by 15 percent in those years, or by about $89,000 per person. Real income in the bottom 90 percent increased by 0.6 percent in those years, or by about $220 per person. The average real income in the bottom 90 percent is only about $33,000 per person, which is a third of the increase achieved by the top 1 percent. Income inequality has many causes, most of which are related to economics, technology, and social organization. Recent economic data suggest improving incomes among the poor and middle class. It will take years to sort out the actual impact of Obamacare on income inequality and on health. See "Income Inequality in the United States," *Inequality.org*, available at http://inequality.org/income-inequality/ (accessed April 15, 2018).

make Americans healthier. Sometimes doctors and hospitals can help people prevent disease and disability, but we now know that most of what doctors and hospitals do is provide treatment and comfort to people after they become ill—when we aren't killing them. And that people build communities and make their own health, as they work together to make democracy stronger.

In 2017, the headlines were all about Trumpcare and about how many people would lose their insurance if it passed. Health policy experts were able to predict how many would lose insurance by how much and how fast premiums would rise once Republicans started to tinker with the health insurance market. Truth be told, many of those predictions were correct. But many of the predictions by people on the right were correct as well. Obamacare is in trouble. Health insurance premiums continue to rise. More insurers will pull out of rural areas unless they are paid well, which means being subsidized by public money, to keep offering their products there. Obamacare works passably in large markets, but it has no cost controls with teeth, so even in large markets health insurance cost continues to rise at 6, 10, or even 15 percent a year, because the drivers of health care cost have nothing to do with health insurance or its reform, which is the dancer but not the dance. Which is not to say the Republicans have any understanding at all of how health insurance markets work or about the remarkably weak relationship between health insurance and public health outcomes. Their doctrinaire approach would have driven costs higher faster and may yet cause health insurance markets to implode.

But the problem with both Obamacare and Trumpcare is that they represent health insurance market reforms, not health care system reforms. Health insurance is the problem, not the solution. The solution is to build a health care system that cares for all Americans, so that we can control cost as we improve the health of the population, which is what a health care system is for.

Obamacare and Trumpcare is what we get when we let other people—government, insurance companies, hospitals, doctors, and other people with something to sell—try to fix it for us. They just figure out how to keep the wealth themselves. Maybe now it's time to see what we get when people and communities try to create a different kind of wealth. Maybe it's time for people and communities to stand up together and make ourselves healthy by fighting for our health care. We'll create health if we do that, because we'll be building community, and health is inseparable from community—and we'll resuscitate democracy in the process.

CHAPTER FIVE

Embers and Sparks:
A Tale of Two or Three Cities, a Couple of States, Two or Three Countries, and a Rural Place or Two

IN CAMDEN, NEW JERSEY, JEFF BRENNER, A DEDICATED FAMILY PHYSICIAN IN solo practice, started to tire out. Brenner cared for a community of the old, the hungry, the tired, and the poor—a population of people on Medicaid and Medicare. He began to wonder why Medicaid couldn't pay him enough to keep his doors open. *These patients of mine keep going to the hospital again and again, and Medicaid keeps paying the hospital, and that costs way more money than I get paid for the work I do,* Dr. Brenner thought. *The work I do, listening to people, taking their phone calls at three in the morning, and seeing them when they are sick is so much more important than what hospitals do when they admit these people again and again. The problems of people in my community—mostly substance use issues and chronic disease—are so much better treated by family doctors in the community.*

Dr. Brenner, as tired as he was, started staying up half the night. He used his computer to analyze data from the hospitals and from Medicaid, and he figured out that huge sums of Medicaid dollars were being spent on people from a few elderly housing developments who didn't have primary care and couldn't get to the doctor. Soon he organized a way to get doctors and nurse practitioners to see them in their homes—and what do you know, Medicaid started spending far less on emergency rooms and hospitalizations for those people, who started living longer and feeling better. (It wasn't so easy or quick to get Medicaid to pay Dr. Brenner better for the care he gave those people, though.) Dr. Brenner won a MacArthur Fellowship for that work and had articles written about him in the medical literature and in the *New Yorker*, and he is trying to help spread his approach across the nation, using teams of doctors, social workers, pharmacists, nurse practitioners, and others.[1]

In San Antonio, Texas, a group of doctors that calls itself WellMed figured out that doctors by themselves weren't that good at taking care of people who were older or had chronic diseases, so they formed teams of people—doctors and nurse practitioners, social workers and pharmacists, and people without health care training they call health coaches—who call or visit the people they take care of regularly, so those people have someone they trust, including health coaches who encourage and remind their patients to do the many complicated tasks needed to keep a chronic disease like diabetes under control. WellMed's doctors care for far fewer patients than most physicians do (six hundred as opposed to two thousand or more) and focus their work on people over sixty-five. Their patients have half the mortality rate of people over sixty-five living in the same state who aren't WellMed patients. They use the hospital only half as much and experience much lower costs.[2]

---

1   Atul Gawande, "The Hot Spotters," *New Yorker*, January 24, 2011, available at https://www.newyorker.com/magazine/2011/01/24/the-hot-spotters (accessed April 30, 2018).

2   R.L. Philips Jr. et al., "Case Study of a Primary Care–Based Accountable Care System Approach to Medical Home Transformation," *Ambulatory Care Management* 34, no. 1 (January–March 2011): 67-77, available at https://journals.lww.com/ambulatorycaremanagement/Abstract/2011/01000/Case_Study_of_a_Primary_Care_Based_Accountable.9.aspx (accessed April 21, 3028). Since this study was published, WellMed was bought by United Health Care and greatly expanded. Time will tell if the approach will remain as effective now that WellMed isn't serving a single community and is controlled by a corporate parent.

In Durham, North Carolina, a community health center noticed a high rate of emergency department visits among its patients who were residents of a large public housing project. The residents of that housing project were elderly, poor, and had many chronic diseases—and many were homebound with little family support. Working with physicians and others from Duke University, that community health center interviewed 350 community residents and discovered that simply assigning a patient to a primary care physician wasn't enough when those people couldn't get to the doctor and struggled with poverty and loneliness. So they put together a team that included local officials, mental health specialists, social workers, community health workers, nutritionists, and occupational therapists, and they used nurse practitioner and physician assistants who went door to door in the housing project, reaching out to every single person. That approach reduced ambulance, emergency room, and hospital costs by 40 percent or more.

The evidence from Camden, San Antonio, and Durham, taken together with a host of other little experiments and demonstrations is pretty clear: you need a team to take care of a population of people, and you need to reach out to the frail and elderly in their homes if you are going to do that affordably and effectively. There is also very strong evidence that our current market, which includes community health centers, doctors' offices, hospitals and hospital emergency departments, urgent care centers, and even retail clinics isn't serving our communities very well, despite how much has been invested in them. The CDC estimates that about 80 percent of people who use emergency departments do so because there is no other place for them to go when they think they need medical attention.[3]

---

3   Renee M. Gindi, Robert A. Cohen, and Whitney K. Kirzinger, "Emergency Room Use among Adults Aged 18–64: Early Release of Estimates from the National Health Interview Survey, January–June 2011," May 2012, available at https://www.cdc.gov/nchs/data/nhis/earlyrelease/emergency_room_use_january-june_2011.pdf (accessed April 15, 2018).

Truth be told, there have been hundreds of attempts to build little health care systems in the U.S. It's a story of embers and sparks: of glowing embers that flare up for a few moments in the wind and send sparks, but until now we haven't had a movement, a wind, that might help the fire catch and create the light and warmth of a health care system serving all Americans.

The earliest actual little health care system experiment I'm aware of began in Mound Bayou, Mississippi, in 1965. Mound Bayou was a community founded 1887 by Isaiah Montgomery and Benjamin Green, former slaves of Jefferson Davis's brother who had migrated from the Davis Bend Plantation to create a self-governing and economically independent African American community. The community thrived at first, and by 1912 had three schools, forty businesses, six churches, a train depot, a newspaper, three cotton gins, a cottonseed oil mill, a zoo, the Carnegie library, a bank, a swimming pool, a sawmill, a Farmers Cooperative and Mercantile company, and a hospital. But Mound Bayou's fortunes declined as the nation changed to an urban, industrialized country, and people left the South for Detroit and Cleveland and Pittsburgh, where there were good jobs and better schools. The population fell from four thousand to less than two thousand. Then the downtown burned in 1948. Owner farmers became sharecroppers, and poverty became widespread. That poverty became more intense in the late 1950s and early 1960s, as effective herbicides, insecticides, chemical fertilizers, and mechanized cotton harvesters replaced the farmworkers and sharecroppers whose livelihoods depended on cotton.

In 1965, Dr. H. Jack Geiger was a civil rights activist turned reporter turned doctor who was a professor at the Harvard University School of Public Health in Boston. As a medical student, Geiger had spent time in South Africa, working at the Phelola Health Center in Natal, a pioneering effort to marry medical services with social and economic organizing—an effort that reflected on the intimate relationship that exists between health, community, the local economy, and local social organization. Dr. Geiger brought home an understanding of the power of these relationships, and in the early 1960s he convinced the Johnson administration, which was just starting its War on Poverty, to fund two community health centers, one urban and one rural, to test the value of these ideas. Dr. Geiger worked with Count Gibson, MD, chair of the Department of Preventative Medicine at Tufts University School of Medicine, who agreed to involve Tufts in this effort.

Geiger had been in the Mississippi Delta with the Medical Committee on Human Rights in the summer of 1964 as part of Freedom Summer, and he returned in late 1965 to find a site for a rural community health center. Mound Bayou appeared to be the place where the need was greatest; it was an overwhelmingly African American community that was suffering desperate rural poverty, and it also had two failing hospitals run by competing African American fraternal organizations that needed support.

What followed was a seven-year experiment in community organizing and health care system design that produced a little health care system. That little health care system addressed itself to the needs of the northern part of Bolivar County, where about ten thousand people lived in five hundred square miles, an area about half the size of Rhode Island. Geiger recruited a community organizer named John Hatch, a Kentucky-born social worker and civil rights activist who was then living in Boston, and who agreed to move back to the segregated South. Hatch traveled the county, meeting its people, learning its customs and culture, learning about its churches and fraternal organizations, and meeting its ministers. He paid careful attention to the lives of people in the most isolated parts of the county, places like Rosedale, Duncan, Round Lake, Marigold, and Alligator, where many people lived in deep poverty on old plantations. At that time, only 29 percent of the population of Bolivar County had running water in their homes, and only 10 percent had flush toilets. Human feces flowed in open drainage ditches that overflowed when it rained.

There was no waste disposal, and people lived in simple shacks that lacked steps and were heated with a single woodstove in the middle of one large room. The Mississippi African American infant mortality rate was 56.2 deaths per thousand live births in 1964, which was more than twice the Mississippi white infant mortality rate—and the highest in the nation.[4] Some people wanted their lives to improve, but many people were afraid—the teachers and the principals and anyone who was on the public payroll served at the pleasure of an all-white school board and had to fear for their jobs. And the small black elite feared for the loss of their positions of leadership in the community.

What John Hatch found was that a desire for medical care wasn't central to the lives of many people in Bolivar County. "Hatch heard about the need for clean water to drink, fuel to heat their shacks, livable housing, pest control, child care and jobs."[5] So Hatch listened. And then he and Geiger adapted their approach to address the needs of the people he was getting to know.

---

4   In 1964, the U.S. infant mortality rate was 21.6 per thousand live births for whites and 41.6 for African Americans; in Mississippi the infant mortality rate was 23.1 per thousand live births for white Mississippians and 56.2 for African American Mississippians. Today the U.S. infant mortality rate is about 6 deaths per thousand live births overall—about 4 deaths per thousand live births for non-Hispanic whites, and about 11 deaths per thousand live births for African Americans. In Mississippi today, there are about 6 deaths per thousand live births for whites and about 11 deaths per thousand live births for whites.

      U.S. Department of Health, Education, and Welfare, "Vital Statistics in the United States 1964, Volume II—Mortality," 2.3 and 2.6, available at https://www.cdc.gov/nchs/data/vsus/mort64_2a.pdf (accessed April 15, 2018); "Infant Mortality by Race," *Kids Count Data Center*, available at http://datacenter.kidscount.org/data/tables/21-infant-mortality-by-race#detailed/2/2-52/false/869,36,868,867,133/10,11,9,12,1,13/285,284 (accessed April 15, 2018).

5   Thomas J. Ward Jr., *Out in the Rural—A Mississippi Health Center and Its War on Poverty* (New York: Oxford University Press, 2016), 43.

Hatch carefully and patiently developed ten health associations in each of ten communities, and out of those associations developed an umbrella organization called the North Bolivar County Health Council, which coordinated the work of the health associations and was able to advise and inform the developing Tufts-Delta Health Center on what the people of Bolivar County really needed and wanted, as well as helping the professionals at the health center understand the challenges and barriers to improving the health of the population and the opportunities that existed. By 1970, the ten health associations had 2,855 members. These people helped the Tufts-Delta Health Center develop its programs, used its programs, and became its ambassadors, helping the communities understand how to use the center and, more importantly, making sure that the health center was serving community needs.

The Tufts-Delta Health Center opened its doors in a temporary space in November 1967, after many attempts—by everyone from the governor of Mississippi to the local black elite—to derail it. Soon it was seeing a hundred people a day.

The health center itself was an extraordinary clinical enterprise. It used a team of physicians, public health nurses, psychologists, social workers, sanitarians, laboratory and X-ray technologists, and others, many of whom were recruited from the community and trained by the health center for their new roles caring for the critically poor community in northern Bolivar County.

What followed was an exceptional period in which Tufts-Delta Health Center, in collaboration with the North Bolivar County Health Council and the ten health associations, worked to improve the lives of thousands of people in northern Bolivar County. When the clinicians at the health center and the members of the health associations recognized that malnutrition was a critical health problem, the clinicians began prescribing food, the best medical treatment for malnutrition, and Dr. Geiger managed to talk the Office of Economic Opportunity into paying for that food. Then the Health Council worked to develop a six-hundred-acre farm co-op that involved over nine hundred families, had six thousand members, employed three hundred people, and distributed fresh and frozen vegetables across northern Bolivar County. When the community and the clinicians identified sanitation as a major health issue, the health center developed an environmental health division. The health center hired Andrew James, the first African American sanitarian in Mississippi, and James and his team roamed the county digging wells, installing sanitary privies, and repairing houses, and, together with the local health associations, helped organize lawsuits and boycotts to give the African American citizens of northern Bolivar County access to the same city water and sewers as the white citizens of northern Bolivar County.

It is hard to know with precision what the public health outcomes of the North Bolivar County Health Council, the health associations, and the Tufts-Delta produced. The whole little health system had unraveled by the end of 1972, as the Nixon administration took apart the Office of Economic Opportunity and the funding for many of these projects dissolved. John Hatch and Andrew James went off to pursue doctorates. Jack Geiger left Tufts to start a new Department of Community Health at Stony Brook University School of Medicine. The farm co-op began growing cash crops instead of fresh fruits and vegetables and by the mid-1970s was absorbed by Alcorn State University as a research farm. The health center, the Health Council, and the local hospital were all consolidated and handed over to local officials to run. By the end of 1972, the health center had stopped functioning as a way to empower communities and improve the lives of everyone in northern Bolivar County, even though it continued to provide clinical services.

There is one anecdotal report that the infant mortality rate in northern Bolivar County dropped in half in the first two years of the health center's operation, but it is difficult to prove the public health impact of the health center's work, given the brief period in which the health center functioned and the population shifts that occurred in Mound Bayou and Bolivar County in the intervening years.[6] The population of Mound Bayou is now half of what it was in 1968. The infant mortality rate in Bolivar County is now among the lowest in Mississippi but still higher than most parts of the U.S.

Looking backward, Dr. Geiger, John Hatch, Andrew James, and others have reflected on the impact the health center had on the lives of the people it touched. Many of those people pursued an education and many more—more than one hundred people from northern Bolivar County—became health professionals, in a place and at a time when few black Mississippians made those choices. Despite difficulties in proving the public health impact, it is hard to believe that the North Bolivar County Health Council, the health associations, and the Tufts-Delta Health Center didn't open the door to democracy to a community of people who had been excluded from the democratic process and the decent life that democracy engenders.

Mound Bayou also served as a model, a standard held up for the rest of the nation to see and rally around. It gave birth to 1,375 other health centers that provide medical care to twenty-five million Americans. Health centers aren't perfect, but they care for the people in their communities who walk through their doors. Their boards are made of 51 percent consumers of their services, but they are selected, not elected, by the communities they serve. They vary in terms of how many primary care services (mental and behavioral health, substance use disorder treatment, emergency medical services, occupational and physical therapy, and nutrition) they offer and in the extent to which they are open evenings and weekends. They don't all take responsibility for the public health of their communities,

---

6   Ward, *Out in the Rural*, 85.

although they are the best organization in each community to do so. But community health center sites exist as public health boots on the ground in nine thousand communities, and they provide us with a starting point, a place to stand, as we prepare to build a health care system for the U.S. From that perspective, Mound Bayou, which gave birth to the community health center, was an unrivaled success.

In Mound Bayou, we learned it's possible to build a little health care system that is run by and for the people it serves, and that by doing so, we can improve the lives of the people in that community and give the people in that community new careers in health care. But we also learned that little health care systems, like small communities, swim in the sea of a larger culture and are unable to protect the integrity of communities by themselves—the integrity of communities is heavily influenced by technology, culture, and the political economy of the nation as a whole.

Another groundbreaking experiment occurred in Hunterdon County, New Jersey, in the years 1946 to 1979.[7] In 1946, Hunterdon County, which is just a few miles west of Princeton, was a little rural county of forty thousand that was populated by (mostly white) chicken farmers, as well as rural American nobility—gentleman farmers with inherited money who liked to foxhunt. The county had an average income lower than the state's average and some pockets of poverty but was also home to some of the state's—and the nation's—wealthiest people. (Hunterdon County now has a population of about 125,000, is much more suburban despite still having many rural areas, and is the fourth-richest county in the nation.) In 1946, the County Board of Agriculture, prompted by three very accomplished women—Rose Angell, director of the Hunterdon County Welfare

---

7   Lloyd B. Westcott, "Hunterdon: The Rise and Fall of a Medical Camelot," *New England Journal of Medicine* 300, no. 17 (April 26, 1979): 952-57.

Board, and Louise Leicester and Ann Stevenson of the County Board of Agriculture—appointed a study committee to explore the feasibility of building a hospital in Hunterdon County. The study committee, which included two of those three women, farmers, businessmen, an auctioneer, and one aging general practitioner, consulted many people and relied heavily on the advice of Lester Evans, MD, of the Commonwealth Fund, which is still a leading voice on health care policy in the U.S., and E.H. Lewinsky-Corwin, PhD, of the New York Academy of Medicine, both of whom had an interest and training in public health as well as medicine. What emerged from the study committee was a report, authored by Lewinsky-Corwin, that proposed "a true community hospital which will be able to provide adequate hospital care to the inhabitants of the county, a health protection service, and a diagnostic service for the convenience of local physicians."[8]

What has been long forgotten is that most hospitals were created to serve the needs of the poor (at a time when people of means who became ill were cared for in their own homes by their personal physicians) or evolved out of the physicians' private practices—a number of early twentieth-century physicians built new wings onto their houses, so that they didn't have to make as many house calls and could make more money in the process. Hunterdon was different from the start, because it evolved out of a community that was looking to design health services for all the people who lived there.

Because its charge was to provide medical services to everyone in the county, the study committee began to imagine a different sort of enterprise, so they called the enterprise a medical center, not a hospital, and designed its little health care system to provide a wide range of "preventive, diagnostic, and

8   A.L. Katcher, *A Time to Remember: Hunterdon County Medical Center—A Health Care Ideal for the People* (Flemington, NJ: Hunterdon Medical Center Foundation, 2003), 62.

restorative services." They built a two-hundred-bed hospital affiliated with NYU–Bellevue Medical Center in Manhattan, which
included fifteen psychiatric beds and a multispecialty clinic with
sixteen different specialties. Hunterdon Medical Center also
provided home health care, outpatient physical therapy and
rehabilitation, child development programs, nutrition and wellness programs, prenatal programs for young parents, a speech
and hearing clinic, and drug and alcohol treatment programs.

But the medical center was really built on the chassis of
primary care. Most medical care was provided by twenty-five
family physicians in private practice spread across the county,
and by four family health centers in more distant parts of the
county, staffed by residents and faculty from one of the first and
best family medicine residency programs in the nation, which
was affiliated with the Rutgers University School of Medicine.[9]
The hospital, the specialists, and the support services functioned
to support the work of the medical center's family physicians.
The specialists functioned as consultants to the family
physicians, and they were prevented by medical center bylaws
from practicing primary care. The county's family physicians
coordinated each person's health care. Each person had a single
physician to go to when they were ill or if they needed advice.

The medical center was a closed shop run by its community. A
special committee of the hospital board, acting on recommendation
of the community and of the medical and administrative staff,
determined which specialties were required and how many

9　Both Mound Bayou and Hunterdon benefited from their academic affili-
　　ations, which brought idealistic young physicians to work in their com-
　　munities and also, perhaps, provided some balance, so that the pressure
　　of daily work and local politics was offset by a larger social context that
　　allowed those young physicians to be nurtured by mission, vision, values,
　　and goals. The medical schools providing the affiliations likely got much
　　more than they gave, because both small health care systems gave pur-
　　pose and meaning to the medicine that medical schools were teaching.

physicians of each specialty to employ. This structure created an ideal environment for patient care and an ideal teaching environment for family medicine residents, who learned from family medicine faculty mentors as they cared for patients and families in their communities and from specialists who were the teachers of and collaborators with their family physician colleagues.

As a result, health care in Hunterdon County remained affordable, with substantially lower rates of emergency and hospital utilization than other parts of the county or even of the earliest HMOs, while its measured public health outcomes remained good. Family physicians were in private practice and billed the patient directly. (This was before health insurance paid for primary care services.) Specialists were all employees of the medical center, which billed patients and insurers for their services.

Hunterdon remained effective and affordable, but only until the mid-1970s, when the specialists objected. Specialists believed that their incomes were being unfairly constrained by this medical staff system, which kept them from having their own patients, from marketing their services to any and all comers, and from having an independent income that they could increase by better marketing and hard work.

There was a two-year period of contention and confrontation, and then a lawsuit and a negotiated settlement—after which the Hunterdon system fell apart. The law was clear. The only thing that matters in our jurisprudence is providing everyone with something to sell equal access to the marketplace. We have no jurisprudence of the common good. The specialists and family physicians started competing with one another for patients. With less work for family physicians, fewer came to practice in Hunterdon County, so there wasn't a family doctor for every person in the county. More people used the emergency department. More people were hospitalized. Costs went up.

Today Hunterdon Medical Center is a pretty good smallish hospital in the middle of New Jersey that has a reasonably good residency program in family medicine but otherwise looks like every other little hospital or medical center in America, with a board and lots of executives who pay themselves high salaries. The county has tripled in population, and lots of the open land has filled in with housing developments and McMansions. Few people remember that the Hunterdon County Medical Center was what a health care system in the United States could have looked like. And while the people of Hunterdon County lost what should have been the flagship health care system in the nation, the people of the United States lost a critical opportunity to see what communities can do to create health care systems for themselves.

Considered together, Roseto, Pennsylvania, Mound Bayou, and Hunterdon County tell us that local culture can have a powerful impact on health, but that impact is easily upended by national and global economic, cultural, and political forces. Whether a little health care system is organized by and from the community, as in Hunterdon County, or whether it is organized from the outside, as Jack Geiger did in Mound Bayou, little health care systems need the support from a larger health care system—from the state and national government—and from the people of the United States, with an understanding that health care is an essential service we need to provide to all Americans.

We need a great wind, a movement, if we are going to build a health care system for the U.S.

Is there a state that does health care better that we can learn from? Not really. In the U.S., states are mostly the same, with some regional variation. The states with the best health outcomes—Massachusetts and California—have cultures that focus, often to the level of obsession, on healthy behaviors and reflect those choices in law and regulation. Massachusetts spends more than almost any other state on health care. California has a health-oriented culture and achieves impressive outcomes, while being one of the lowest-spending states in the country, so likely deserves more public health attention than it gets.[10]

The states with the worst health outcomes—Mississippi, Alabama, Louisiana, West Virginia, and Arkansas—are old slave states that have remained poor and that still struggle with the legacy of racial divides. Interestingly, white citizens of these states generally have worse health outcomes than white citizens in the rest of the U.S., although their health outcomes are generally somewhat better than the health outcomes of their African American neighbors. Their health care spending varies— West Virginia is twelfth-highest, Louisiana is right smack in the middle, and Mississippi, Alabama, and Arkansas rank on the low side of average spending nationally, although all of the poor outcome states except Arkansas spend more than California.

So culture matters. Maybe it matters more than money. Certainly it matters more than medical care.

There is one state program that is worth calling out in this discussion, as we think about what works for states. In Rhode Island, there is something called a universal vaccine purchasing program. The state lifts money from each health insurance contract, a certain amount of money for each person, and puts that money into a vaccine purchasing pool. Rhode Island then buys all the vaccine we need for every person in the state and supplies that vaccine at no charge to doctors, health centers, pharmacies, hospitals, home health organizations, mass vaccinators,

---

10 "List of U.S. State and Territories by Life Expectancy," *Wikipedia,* available at https://en.wikipedia.org/wiki/List_of_U.S._states_by_life_expectancy (accessed April 15, 2018); "Infant mortality rate in the United States as of 2017, by state (deaths per 1,000 live births)," *Statista,* available at https://www.statista.com/statistics/252064/us-infant-mortality-rate-by-ethnicity-2011/ (accessed April 15, 2018); "Health Care Expenditures per Capita by State of Residence," *KFF,* available at http://kff.org/other/state-indicator/health-spending-per-capita/?currentTimeframe=0 (accessed April 15, 2016).

and nursing homes, and those people and organizations run around the state getting everyone vaccinated. We have clinics in high schools, town halls, and shopping malls in every corner of the state. Because we buy vaccine in bulk, we save 15 percent, and because we have a single process, our vaccinators don't have to try to game the market and aren't flummoxed by that market, which can get tricky and aggressive for a single medical practice that must buy vaccine for large numbers of people at once. So the vaccine program remains relatively affordable, despite attempts by vaccine manufacturers to bid up the price. As a result, Rhode Island has had the best vaccination rates in the nation for a number of years.

So states can matter, if they put public health first and design organized, intelligent processes that recognize the problems caused by our medical products and pharmaceutical market and design programs that benefit everyone—programs that push back against the market and focus on achieving the best health for all their residents.

But other countries provide the most insight into what health care systems are and can be. For years there have been public health rumors about other countries having health care systems that work better than our market. They say there is a primary care doctors on every block in Cuba, and the Cubans have low costs, little infant mortality, and long life expectancy, despite the U.S. blockade. I got to spend time with physicians and nurses from around the world in Nicaragua in the 1980s and heard stories about very low caesarian section rates in the Netherlands and smarter asthma treatment in East Germany and Scandinavia. In Spain, they developed a network of primary care centers and reduced costs by 15 percent. Denmark developed an (all-private) primary care system that has allowed the Danes to close more than half of their hospitals (almost all public), decreasing hospital utilization by 40 percent and controlling costs—and they continue to be one of the healthiest countries in the world.[11]

Still, it is hard to find a country similar enough to the U.S. to make a good comparison. We are more diverse than most places, we have more guns than most places, we have a surprisingly high birth rate, significant income inequality, lots more drug and alcohol use, and, until recently, we had much more immigration than most other countries in the world. Many of our children grow up in poverty, which makes us different from the rest of the developed world. A few recent books have compared the health insurance schemes of different countries and what it is like to be sick in other countries—but no one has ever looked at the best health care systems in the world, the systems that produce the best public health and do so at the lowest cost, to see what they have in common.

From the perspective of public health and affordability, Luxembourg, Norway, Finland, and Iceland have the most effective health care systems in the world. These are hard countries to compare to the U.S.: they are monochromatic, not socially or genetically diverse, and have cold climates that aren't like the climate in the U.S. Still, they have infant mortality rates that are about one-third of what our infant mortality rate is, life expectancies that are three or four years longer than the life expectancy in the U.S., and health care costs that are about a third of ours. But these countries are so different from the U.S. that no comparison of health care systems seemed reasonable.

I was about to abandon this line of inquiry when a little light bulb went off in my head. Once upon a time, Finland, and particularly a far eastern province called North Karelia, had the highest rate of heart disease and heart disease death in the world. Finland used to be the poster child for what happens when you put together a sedentary lifestyle with a diet heavy in meat and simple carbohydrates. Drug companies that made cholesterol-lowering

---

11 Gawande, "The Hot Spotters."

drugs used to flock to Finland to test their drugs, so most of the early reports about how to prevent heart disease that appeared in the medical literature had lead authors with long funny-sounding Finnish names that made them seem extra authentic.

And then the rate of heart disease in some parts of Finland dropped by 80 percent.

So what happened? How did Finland go from having the worst cardiovascular illness and mortality in the world to having one of the longest life expectancies in the world?

Maybe Finland deserved another look.

It turns out that two interesting things happened in Finland. First, the Finns took a creative approach to helping people change their diets and get more exercise. Then they built a health care system.

In 1972, the Finnish Ministry of Health sent a young public health physician named Pekka Puska to North Karelia and charged him with reducing the rate of heart disease in that province.[12] Puska understood that it was better to prevent disease than to try to cure it after the damage had been done and that doctors and hospitals were no better at preventing disease than trucked-in food supplies were at preventing famine. So Puska took a different approach. He and his team began to involve communities directly in changing their diets and in helping people get regular exercise. They involved women's organizations; they gave afternoon "longevity parties," explaining the role of diet and exercise in preventing heart disease; they gave out recipe books and recruited over 1,500 lay ambassadors to tell their friends and the community

---

12   Dan Buettner, "The Finnish Town That Went on a Diet," *Atlantic*, April 7, 2015, available at http://www.theatlantic.com/health/archive/2015/04/finlands-radical-heart-health-transformation/389766/ (accessed April 15, 2018); "Fat to Fit: How Finland Did It," *Guardian*, January 15, 2005, available at https://www.theguardian.com/befit/story/0,15652,1385645,00.html (accessed April 15, 2018).

organizations with which they were involved about how to live a heart-healthy life. But the team didn't stop there. They began to work with food producers and helped to create rural co-ops (like Jack Geiger in Mound Bayou) that turned land used for dairy farming into land used to produce and then freeze fresh berries, which Finns love. Then they worked with grocers, who now feature those fresh and frozen berries. Then they worked with sausage makers and got them to replace the fat and salt in the pork sausages that are a staple of the North Karelian diet with mushrooms. At the same time, they worked on smoking, getting local governments to make workplaces and public buildings smoke-free and starting smoking cessation contests, challenging villages to compete over how many people in each one quit. Then they began to work on promoting physical activity. Local governments got money to build exercise facilities—swimming pools, ballparks, and snow parks for cross-country skiing. Then Puska's team began to invade the local pubs. They began to work with the (mostly middle-aged) men who occupied the barstools and the tables. Those men were lent bicycles, taken on walking and biking tours, and involved in team sports. Doctors began to prescribe exercise the way they used to prescribe medication for high blood pressure and high cholesterol, and soon everyone realized that diet and exercise were more effective than medication. And all those biking tours and the cross-country ski touring turned out to help the local economy, as well as bringing people back in contact with one another. It took ten years of focus on exercise, but now the whole county is exercising—and men can expect to live seven years longer and women six years longer than they did in 1972.

Starting in 1972, the Finns also began to change their health care system. They organized a health care system composed of municipal health centers, each serving ten thousand people, that provide clinical medicine and dentistry, public health and prevention, home care, and even basic inpatient care to all the people who live in each municipality.[13] "Health centres offer a wide variety of services: outpatient medical care, inpatient care in inpatient wards (in larger cities these can be classified more as a general practitioner [GP] run hospitals), preventive services, dental care, maternity care, child health care, school health care, care for older people, family planning, physiotherapy and occupational health care. . . . Health centres are usually well equipped with staff and medical technologies. In addition to the physicians' and nurses' consulting rooms, there are normally X-ray facilities, a clinical laboratory, facilities for minor surgery and endoscopic examinations and equipment such as electrocardiogram and ultrasound."[14]

There is little strange or interesting about the Finnish system, except that it exactly mirrors the description of a health care system that follows in Chapter Seven, a description that was based on the best health policy science available. It isn't possible to know how much the Finnish municipal health center system contributes to Finland's health outcomes, which result from many social and cultural factors as well as health care system design. But it is more than a little interesting that such a system exists in a nation that had the worst heart disease mortality in the world forty years ago yet now has among the best public health outcomes in the world and delivers those outcomes at less than half of what Americans pay for our disordered health care in our disordered market.

---

13 This system appears to combine the U.S. version of nursing homes with the U.S. version of community hospitals. It is a very clever approach that leverages the infrastructure of nursing homes, which have to supply round the clock nursing, and expands what nursing homes do, so they can provide the kind of short-term hospital-level care that community hospitals (which are disappearing in the U.S. because of changes in technology that has made many of them unnecessary) now provide.

14 European Observatory on Health Systems and Policies, "Health Systems in Transition (HiT) profile of Finland," *Health Systems and Policy Monitor*, available at http://www.hspm.org/countries/finland21082013/livinghit.aspx?Section=6.3%20Primary%20/%20ambulatory%20care&Type=Section (accessed April 16, 2018).

CHAPTER SIX

What Our Health Care System Could and Should Look Like If We Want This Democracy to Hold

WHAT WOULD OUR WORLD LOOK LIKE IF WE SPENT $3 TRILLION STRENGTHENING democracy instead of enriching individuals and corporations? What would our $3 trillion spend look like if we were trying to use that money to improve the public's health?

In a health care system, every community of ten thousand people would have a primary care center able to provide 90 percent of the health services every person in that community needs. In small towns that are more than ten miles away from one of these primary care centers, every community of a thousand people would have a one-clinician office that would be linked to a primary care center or five to ten other small offices, so they together could offer 90 percent of the health services every person needs. The health services provided by these primary care centers would include physical, mental and behavioral, and dental care provided by internists, pediatricians, family physicians, dentists, oral hygienists, nurse practitioners, physician assistants, nurse midwives, substance abuse counselors, social workers, psychologists, nutritionists, physical therapists, emergency medical technicians, and others. Those primary care centers would be open from 8:00 a.m. to 8:00 p.m. every weekday and from 9:00 a.m. to 5:00 p.m. on weekends. The primary care centers would also be responsible for maintaining and improving the health of each community. They would know everyone in each community and would make sure every person has access to the prevention they need when they need it. They would be charged with keeping the entire population of that community up to date on vaccinations, colonoscopies, mammograms, and pap smears, and with coaching the people who are at greatest risk to stop smoking and get into recovery and helping them lose weight and exercise.

Every ten of these primary care practices would be affiliated with a multiclinic, where specialists would be available to see patients and consult with primary care clinicians, and every ten multiclinics would be affiliated with a community hospital. Every ten community hospitals would be affiliated with a regional hospital, and all regional hospitals would be affiliated with a network of national specialty hospitals dedicated to research about and treatment of specific diseases and conditions. All these hospitals would be publicly funded. Private practice specialists and private hospitals would continue to function as they do now, funded by a system of private insurance, which would be available for purchase by people who want to opt out of the public system. But because the bulk of services would be publicly funded, this private system would comprise no more than 10 percent of all health care expenditures, and so insurance companies would shrink to a fraction of their current size—and their lobbying money and political leverage would shrink as well. The private and public care systems could exist in a dynamic balance, each providing competition for the other. That competition might provide people with a choice and might drive each system to continuously improve.

If we had a real health care system like that we'd spend $2 trillion a year—not $3 trillion. We'd need to accommodate the massive unemployment of midlevel bureaucrats and administrators, all of who are employed now only because the market that we have is so wasteful. But they could all go to work installing ꜱolar collectors on roofs, growing food locally, building safe and affordable housing, running public transportation, building libraries, running Ys and community centers, and teaching our kids, all of which could be done for $1 trillion.

What would it be like to use a primary care center? First, you could choose you own doctor and dentist from the twenty or so clinicians who would work at each primary care center. For routine care—scheduled physical examinations, follow-up visits, dental cleanings, and the like—the primary care center would function much like most medical and dental offices do today, only the center would be close to your house and more likely to provide open hours that reflect your needs. A larger staff means that the center's professionals can flex hours and each provide services at times primary care and dental practices are not now usually open. The clinicians are likely to know you, your family, and your neighbors, because most of those people will also use the center and will be aware of what's available in your community. X-rays, labs, medications, counseling, substance use disorder treatment, recovery support, and occupational and physical therapy would all be available at the center, which would make your visits exceptionally efficient.

If you are sick, the center will be able to see you that day, and all you will need to do is walk in, rather than spend time on the telephone waiting for an appointment. Most of the time you'll be seen by your own doctor, but sometimes you'll see one of your doctor's associates, who will tell your doctor about the visit. If you turn out to be sick enough to need the hospital, an ambulance staffed by center personal will take you there. Your doctor will call the hospital, so the hospital will know you are coming, and your medical record will be available to the hospital, so they know all about you. Your doctor will be able to look at your hospital record every day you are there, will be fully briefed about your stay, and thus will be ready to work with you the moment you are discharged. When you are ready to be discharged, a team of center staff will come to your house to make sure things are ready for you, and once you are home, you'll get daily visits from a home health nurse and from nursing assistants to make sure you are comfortable and that everything is progressing as expected.

If you are too sick to come to the center, the center ambulance, staffed by emergency medical technicians, will come to your house, quickly evaluate your situation, call your doctor, and together with your doctor decide what to do next: the hospital by ambulance, the center for an urgent evaluation, a visit from the home health team, or a ride on a Life Flight helicopter. These decisions will be made after consulting you, understanding what you want and need, and after a quick discussion with the clinician who knows you and your family best.

What if you need services that the center doesn't provide? What if you need chemotherapy, hip replacement surgery, have an obscure genetic disorder that requires special foods, or develop a heart problem? In that case, your doctor will be able to work with the specialists at the multiclinic and the regional hospital, and together with you work out the best plan of care. Perhaps the multiclinic will have what you need. Perhaps you'll need to go to a national specialty hospital. Regardless of the choice, the center's staff will work with and for you, making sure you get to the right place quickly.

What if you don't want to have anything to do with doctors? Folks from the center will try to check in with you once or twice a year, just to see how you are. They'll call or come by to see if there is anything you need. They'll walk through the neighborhood's churches and mosques, farmers' markets and grocery stores, hairdressers and barbers, and bars and nightclubs, checking in, giving flu shots in the fall, giving you coupons or other opportunities to get you exercising, asking you to come along on bike rides or hikes or join in dance nights that they have organized with the city's parks and rec department, reminding people to get tested for HIV, hepatitis C, and cholesterol, teaching about tasty food that is inexpensive and nutritious, and helping the remaining smokers to quit. The center will do its best to keep track of everyone in the community, to make sure everyone knows the correct steps to take to address preventable disease and has access to the health services they want.

There it is. That's what a health care system looks like. Scary that it is so simple. Scary that we are already paying for it and that moving to a rational system would cost us a trillion dollars less—and that despite all the fearmongering this doesn't involve some massive new investment of funds for venture capitalists to play with. Scarier yet is that all the moving parts—the primary care clinicians and practices, the specialty groups, and the hospitals—are already in place but have never been organized into a system that provides health care to all Americans. We have too many hospitals and too few primary care practices, but changing those ratios is much easier than changing our politics and our ideology, which is what has brought us to the ridiculous place we now occupy in regard to our health and health care.

The design of a health care system that exists to strengthen democracy is easy. The politics that prevent us from getting there are incredibly complex. Too many people, making too much money, stand in the way of the United States creating a health care system that is personal, rational, equal, and just.

Change is scary and complex.

The health care market won't change easily. The Affordable Care Act taught us that. Vested interests will fight tooth and nail to keep things as they are. They will lie, cheat, steal, and threaten us all with death.

Nothing will change unless we act up. The likelihood of success is small. But the likelihood of success without trying is zero.

If you look honestly at the presidential campaign of 2016, you'll see where we are and where we are going if we don't act up. Our democracy is slipping away. And there is no one to blame. Democracy happens when we act up. That's what democracy is, and a political revolution in health care is both democracy in action and exactly how we can bring democracy back to life.

CHAPTER SEVEN

How Can We Get from Here to There?
How to Create a Political Revolution in Health

MAKE NO MISTAKE. CHANGING A $3.2 TRILLION INDUSTRY INTO A HEALTH CARE system for all Americans is a huge undertaking. It will take ten to twenty years and the work of millions of people—a movement, not a campaign. We know from the 1993 attempt to reform health insurance and from the Affordable Care Act that the health care profiteers and their affiliated bureaucracy will do everything in their power to prevent us from having a health care system—fake news, personal attacks, disinformation campaigns, perhaps even intimidation and threats of violence. But we also know from our history that Americans *can* change our society, because we have done that many times before, which is what makes the U.S. forever interesting and vital. We rejected colonialism and embraced democracy, ended slavery, gave women the right to vote, used the labor union movement to protect the lives of working people, ended legal segregation (more or less), ended the Vietnam War, pushed the world to contain the nuclear arms race (more or less), and created marriage equality. Revolt is central to our identity. Our ability to collaborate in the face of danger is part of what has allowed this nation to succeed.

To create a health care system for the United States, we'll need a presence in every American community—and we'll need a national coordinating council. Local chapters, if you will, are necessary to help Americans understand what's wrong and how to fix it and start building small health care systems to care for their own communities. We'll create a national coordinating council made up of organizations that already have members in many communities, organizations with expertise in the health professions and those that represent small businesses and the labor union movement or that are concerned with the public health. The national council is necessary to create trenchant messaging, so that we involve all Americans in this process and have a powerful advocate in every state legislature and in Congress, which will allow us to write and pass enabling legislation to give the U.S. health care system the breadth and depth it needs to care for all of us.

The Movement for Health Care in America will have four aspects. We'll expose and educate. We'll mobilize health care workers. We'll organize small health care systems in every community. And we'll build a national political movement—a political revolution in health care—to pass enabling legislation at the state and local level. Which means we have to organize ourselves, act up, and reorganize what we already have, so that we take care of *all* Americans.

The Movement for Health Care in America starts with people who know something is wrong: people who pay for health care; patients and purchasers of insurance; the small businesses and large businesses now struggling with health care cost; health care professionals and health care workers who are not professionals.

We'll walk on two legs—organizing health care workers and health professionals to revolt and organizing people who want affordable, coherent health care to build little health care systems in their own communities. We'll show health care workers who is industrializing their professional lives and how much money the health care profiteers are making by doing that. We'll show the people who are now paying for health care just how much money is being stolen from them, who is taking it, and how. Then we'll show them what a health care system looks like and describe how much money it will save and how we can have healthier people for a fraction of the money we are now spending.

Here are the steps we'll follow:

Expose and Educate

People who are patients and businesses that pay the freight have to talk over and over again about how much money is being taken from them and what they could do with that money if it wasn't being taken. Health insurance costs $11,000 per person per year. Other countries with better health outcomes pay $2,500 to $4,000 per year. Family health insurance now costs $25,000 to $30,000 per year. That's twice what it's worth. So every family is giving up $12,500 to $15,000 every year—the price of a new car every year or the money it costs for people to pay their mortgage if they own their own home. Which is why more people don't own homes, and perhaps even why some people are homeless. The public money we should have been spending on affordable housing is being diverted to pay for health insurance that's too expensive. Insurance pays for products and services we don't really need and creates profits for the health care profiteers, who eat us out of house and home. We need to say that over and over again, until everyone understands.

We'll show people how health insurance represents wage theft. When health insurance companies raise rates 6 or 10 or 15 percent a year, that's money your employer can't put into raises for you, which means the money for higher insurance premiums is money coming out of your pocket. It would be one thing if that money went to make us all healthier, but life expectancy in the U.S. is falling, not rising. Life expectancy is falling because too many of us are getting high, drinking, or committing suicide, choices people make when they are desperate, when they have no future, which is exactly what happens when someone (the health care profiteers?) takes the value of their work from them in ways they can sense but not clearly see. More money spent on health care can't make anyone better off. Only a fair political system, an economy that lets us share the wealth, people getting high less, drinking less, smoking less, and public spending that builds and runs better schools, builds safe housing, improves public transportation, and invests in communities and community development can do that.

We'll show how health insurance and health care costs hurt America's small and large businesses and stifle the American economy. If those businesses could buy health insurance for what the health care it provides is actually worth, our businesses could price their products competitively and sell more products here and abroad. Then both our economy *and* our stock market would boom, and we'd have jobs here, instead of sending them to Mexico and Southeast Asia (where health care costs a small fraction of what it costs here).

We'll say over and over again that it's the cost of health care and *not* illegal immigration that is stealing American jobs and constraining our prosperity. We'll remind people every chance we get that the health care profiteers steal from us in four different ways—once when they take actual money out of our actual pockets, a second time when the loss of buying power slows growth in the domestic economy, a third time when the loss of price competitiveness slows growth in international trade, and a fourth time when they divert the public money that should be going to education, housing, public transportation, and community development, instead creating profit for themselves.

We'll follow the money and show others where the money trail leads. It's time to out the executives of so-called nonprofit organizations who make $400,000 a year or more, starting with those who are making million-dollar salaries from the medical market, while the average annual wage in the U.S. hovers around

$45,000 a year. It's time we outed the health professionals, the doctors, and the health care lawyers who are making that kind of money. It's time to out the pharmaceutical companies who take five-dollar drugs, manipulate the law and the market, and sell them for $1,500 or more, mostly of public money, and it's time to out the politicians and labor leaders and others who are taking bribes to enable health care profiteering one way or another.

We'll show how health care cost inflation cannibalizes the body politic. In little Rhode Island, we spend $12 billion a year on health care. At 6 percent inflation in health care expense, that means our health care costs go up $720 million a year. That money, if we could capture it, is equivalent to the salaries of twelve thousand teachers, and there are only sixteen thousand public school teachers in the whole state. Or that money, if we could capture it, would buy us 2,880 units of affordable housing, enough to house thirteen thousand people. There are four thousand people homeless in Rhode Island each year, so we could house them all, with enough money left over to pay the salaries of eight thousand new teachers, if that was how we wanted to spend it. And that's only the cost of health care inflation. The bill for all the money that's wasted—or pulled off as profit for health care profiteers—is around $4-6 billion a year, and that's only in little Rhode Island. We'll run this analysis for every state and every city and town, because the numbers are overwhelming. Every community of ten thousand people is spending $100 million a year on health care. That's more than each community spends on its roads, its police and fire protection, its water and its sewage, and its schools combined. The money we waste on health care profiteering, unnecessary care, and fraud is enough to send the all the kids of that community to a four-year college and graduate school for free and liberate generations from mountains of immoral educational debt. That's the information we will expose, and that's why it is reasonable to expect that our neighbors and communities will join us in revolting.

We have to get and post hospital administrator salaries, health insurance company executive salaries, doctors' salaries, nursing salaries, and even the salaries of the janitors, the certified nursing assistants, the medical assistants, and the home health aides, and then we'll be ready to talk knowledgeably about health care company profits. We'll have to get, know, and spread the numbers on the injuries and deaths the medical services marketplace causes every year. Then we'll have to change how we talk about health care. We should never say "health care system" again, because no health care system exists in the United States. Instead, when we talk about health care, we should only say "wealth extraction system" or "medical services marketplace," so that we start telling one another the truth about what we've got. We'll need to inject language about costs and profit into everything we say about health care, again and again, until people see what is, instead of what is being sold to them. We should never say, for example, "Go down to CVS and pick up a couple of Advil." Instead, we should say, "Go down to CVS, a company that made $5.2 billion in profit in 2015 and whose CEO Larry Merlo made $12.1 million that year, and pay five to ten dollars for a couple of Advil, so that Larry Merlo can get his $12.1 million plus bonus and so that all those shareholders get paid." We should never say, "Go down to Man's Best Hospital to get your abdominal aortic aneurysm fixed." Instead, we should say, "An abdominal aortic aneurysm is a scary and dangerous thing. The risk of rupture and your dying from it is 5 percent per year. The surgery can be lifesaving, but the risk of *not* dying from it is 95 percent a year, the risk of a major complication is 10 to 20 percent, and the risk of getting an infection just from being in that hospital is 5 percent. And, by the way, the hospital CEO makes $3 million a year and gets a bonus based on the financial performance of the hospital, so don't be surprised that everyone at the hospital is pushing you to have the surgery. It's in the hospital CEO's interest and the surgeon's interest, and even in the nurses' interest to make sure that Man's Best Hospital does as many surgeries as possible, and also to make sure that not one extra penny is wasted on your comfort or your safety. But *you* are in charge of your own health, and you shouldn't ever listen to someone who is or might profit from your choice. Not ever."

We'll show how advertising has been used to create a culture in which health care profiteering has become morally acceptable. The health care profiteers and their medical services market showers billions of messages onto our screens, radio programming, and billboards each year—something like $50-100 billion of advertising, much of which is devoted to getting us to do something that makes them richer but harms us. Pharmaceutical company advertising, hospital advertising, food product advertising, cigarette advertising, alcohol advertising, gun manufacturer advertising, and even the advertising for those cool little scooters that people with disabilities drive at the side of the road—it all legitimizes the wealth extraction that we have built the health care market around, and none of it helps us build a common life.

Drug company advertising in particular contains the very strong implicit message that you don't need a health care system to shift through mounds of technical evidence that helps us understand who in the population needs what; that instead, you can make your own decision, as a consumer, instead of as a citizen. Every time a drug company ad says consult your doctor, they are saying that you ought to drive your own decisions about what you want as a consumer, that it isn't necessary for there to be a health care system out there that makes sure that everyone who needs a medicine or a vaccine gets the medicine or vaccine they actually need.

Notice that there is no medical services counter-advertising, which is what we used to do to try to counteract cigarette company advertising. If we had it, medical services counter-advertising would be saying that lots of medicines are used unnecessarily, increasing the cost of health insurance, and that many medicines have side effects that become more meaningful when they aren't really needed, and those side effects contribute to the 250,000 deaths a year in the U.S. from medical accidents and misadventures. No one is putting pictures of people injured by medical misadventures on TV, or of obese people with diabetes and heart disease who ate the industrial food goop that the advertisers told them to buy. And it is hard to show pictures of the schools and public transportation and community centers we don't have. So we'll have to start talking about those schools and that public transportation and community centers, because talking with one another is the best way we have of counteracting the advertisements that the health care profiteers are able to buy. And we know that talking with other people works best when hundreds of thousands of us do it together.

Every time a hospital or specialty group advertises on billboards, on the radio, or on TV, they are working to convince you that there is no need for a health care system—that the service they sell is adequate and will keep you safe. There is no real counter-advertising to hospital advertising either, and most of us believe what we hear, particularly when we hear it over and over again. We need to be saying that we have twice the number of hospitals we need, and those hospitals cost us money, make executives and specialists rich, but contribute nothing to the public's health or to our common life, other than keeping a huge number of people employed. Then we need to be saying that the same people could be doing something productive for society, instead of working in a process that is destructive to democracy.

Along the way, we need to help our fellow citizens learn about the $500 million a year the medical industrial complex spends on lobbying. Let's find and list that spending, company by company, state by state, and legislator by legislator, so that all Americans can see for themselves how the business of medicine works.

We have to talk about the profits in real dollars of for-profit hospitals, drug companies, and insurance plans. We have to tell people over and over again about the way drug companies run by venture capitalists have made generic drugs private and inflated prices a thousandfold and how the public process, proposed and voted on by our senators and members of congress, let this happen. How those drug companies and the other health care profiteers spend $500 million a year on lobbying those senators and members of congress and how much money each of those politicians is taking from the various health care profiteers. We have to talk about the $1 trillion a year that is wasted and should be used for education, housing, community centers, and safe streets. And we'll keep talking about that $1 trillion until we have a health care system that isn't wasting so much money and destroying our dignity and our common life.

This information is widely available, but it has been invisible because no one is making it a part of our public culture. The civil rights movement and now Black Lives Matter have shown us the racism that has always been with us. Those movements helped us understand how racism has its grip on the throat of our culture, so that we could see and start to confront the racism in ourselves, our culture, and the nation. Occupy helped us understand income inequality and how it is destroying democracy. We have a medical services market, not a health care system. That market is stealing form all of us and making the rich richer. The health care profiteers are robbing us blind. Everyone has to know.

Perhaps our greatest challenge is to show Americans what a real health care system looks like. A real health care system includes all Americans and provides each of us with health care services—prevention, diagnosis, treatment, and cure—in our communities, schools, and workplaces. A real health care system keeps us healthy enough to put our ideals into practice—one nation, indivisible, with liberty and justice for all—and so allows us all to pursue happiness, individually and together. A real health care system builds our identity as one people who have used our freedom to care for one another, keeping us equal enough to live as free individuals who are part of a free people.

We'll help everyone understand what a real health care system is and how it works, and then make sure everyone knows how a real health care system saves lives, makes communities healthier, improves our personal experience of health care services, and saves money, all at the same time.

First, we'll tell Americans about the effective components of a health care system we already have. We already have 1,375 community health centers that provide the best measured primary care to twenty-five million Americans at nine thousand different sites, health care that is for people, not for profit, places where you get health care regardless of your ability to pay. We already have a great EMS system in most communities that respond to emergencies, regardless of your ability to pay. We already have many nonprofit hospitals that serve most communities, even though those hospitals sometimes forget that their mission is to help us improve the health of all Americans. These hospitals, because of federal legislation passed a half century ago and reinforced with other federal legislation passed a quarter century ago, serve all Americans who need urgent care regardless of their ability to pay, even though they have learned to enrich their executives and their specialists while providing the care the law requires. We already have a few nonprofit HMOs that are learning to organize and manage care, even if they are way too expensive because of the competitive nature of the health insurance marketplace. And we already have a quarter to a half million or more primary care clinicians practicing in every city and town in the U.S., working overtime to bring this essential service to most Americans—and doing that in the face of a medical services and insurance marketplace that has devalued the relationships primary care clinicians try to build with patients and stripped them of needed resources.

Then we'll tell people what other countries do and how they do it. We'll talk about Finland, Norway, Ireland, Singapore, Costa Rica, Cuba, Portugal, the UK, Spain, Canada, and France—places where everyone has health care in their own communities, where the cost is a fraction of what Americans pay and the services and outcomes are far better. We'll talk about the visiting nurses in the UK, who check in on every new baby every day for a month; about the community health centers in Finland, where there is one for every ten thousand people; about Cuba, where there is a doctor on every city block; and about Spain and Portugal, where every person has access to primary health care.

And finally, we will show people the cost projections: how we can have better health and better health care if we reorganize our existing services into a system that provides services to all Americans, how instead of a market where costs rise 6 percent or more every year, we'll have better services, closer to home, and pay only two-thirds of what we pay now, saving, as a nation, $500 billion to $1 trillion a year.

It will take a mass movement to spread this information. We'll need to mobilize health care workers and communities to reach all Americans.

We need lectures and conversations and teach-ins. We need to get this information to every city council, chamber of commerce, Rotary Club, church, synagogue, mosque, adult education program, and every grand rounds in every community hospital in these United States. It will take a hundred thousand people to give these talks, but the only way to fix this mess, whether we like it or not, is for a hundred thousand of us volunteer.

And we have lots of educating to do.

No one in the U.S. has ever seen a health care system, but lots of people and organizations do everything they can to frighten us and our neighbors. The moment we begin to talk about changing just the insurance system, the scaremongers appear. "You'll lose your choice of doctors!" they scream. "You don't want the government running your health care! You'll destabilize the health insurance market! There will be death panels deciding who shall live and who shall die!"

They won't mention that the choice of doctors is already limited by cost, income, and location. They won't mention that the health insurance market is already destabilizing the lives of many Americans and propping itself up with lobbyists' bribes. They won't mention that the death panels already exist—they are the stockholders of pharmaceutical companies and the medical directors of health insurance companies. Try going to see an orthopedist in the U.S. if you have Medicaid or, even worse, no insurance. Before they will see you, many specialists require you to sign away your rights to contest your bill or sue them for any reason and to commit to paying for *their* legal costs if you have a legal dispute. Try getting an expensive, lifesaving, name-brand drug if you don't have health insurance—and sometimes even if you do. If you don't have health insurance, tough luck. If you do have health insurance, get ready to be put through the mill, as your insurance company throws up every roadblock it can think of to avoid paying for what you need, which they think costs them too much. Along the way, no one questions why it is this way, why we don't make drugs cheaply and give them out for free—something we could do in a world in which health care is for people, not for profit. In a world where democracy matters.

In fact, no one knows how a well-designed health care system would impact the choice of doctors. It is very possible we could *increase* the choice of doctors or hospitals—but there is no one taking out advertisements saying *that* on TV.

Along the way, we need to remind everyone that the government supplies us with clean water to drink, provides fire and police protection, educates our kids, and delivers the mail.

We need to remind everyone that no one says to watch out for socialism in the fire department or in the police department. We need to remind everyone that the people who serve all of us are heroes, which is exactly how we should and will think of health care workers again once we've found the courage to stand up and make health care nonprofit, so it serves the common good and not the health care profiteers.

We need to educate ourselves about some basic health care facts, and then educate others, if we are going to build a health care system for the U.S. and strengthen democracy.

We can build a health care system for the U.S. that includes everyone, actually improves our health, and saves us a trillion dollars a year. Learn about it. That's the message we'll be spreading, until every American knows this inconvenient truth.

Mobilize Health Care Workers, Revolt, March, Agitate, Boycott, Strike, Occupy CMS

One of the many unintended consequences of health care profiteering is its impact on health care workers and our professionalism. Health care workers all across the U.S. have experienced thirty years of speedups and industrialization. Once upon a time, we were health professionals committed to unself-interested advocacy, to putting the health and safety of patients and their communities first. Now we are cost centers, commodities that (no longer "who") reduce profit by costing the profiteers money when we spend time listening to patients, sitting on a bedside, holding a cool compress to someone's forehead, or changing a bed so the person in it has cool, comfortable sheets to sleep on. We are now measured every six ways from Sunday. Our quality is continuously checked on and improved. Our patient satisfaction scores are continually monitored. Our productivity (productivity! in professions that exist to listen to patients!) is computed and compared to that of our colleagues and to national benchmarks. As a result, many of us feel tired out, used up, and heartbroken, because the work lives we have aren't what we want and we aren't doing anything like the work we went into the health professions to do. We are well paid, but many of us do everything we can to reduce our hours, because the money is only barely worth the pain, and many more of us retire early, so we can sit home and wonder about how we allowed the health care enterprise, which was once about helping, not selling, to get away from us and from our communities.

The conditions for health care workers differ market by market. In Boston people are well paid, but their electronic medical records have made their lives hell. New York has strong unions, but its workforce is too small to handle the volume. In Memphis specialists do well, but there aren't enough primary care clinicians, so emergency rooms are overburdened. In Dallas the non-professional staff is poorly paid and not organized, so patients have trouble moving from place to place inside hospitals, and lab and X-ray services are slow and unreliable. These local challenges have made health care institutions fertile ground for organizing, and tapping into health care worker discontent is a crucial strategy that the Movement for Health Care in America will use. Once health care workers find the courage to confront the alienation in their professional lives, they will discover that they have the responsibility to support and the ability to lead the movement to build a health care system for the U.S.

We'll use organizers in every market, focused on what health care workers in each place want most to change. The opportunity here is to organize across professional boundaries, to bring physicians together with nurses, occupational therapists, X-ray techs, and porters, creating powerful organizations of people who know their professions and are empowered to take the institutions that employ them back from the profiteers. One added advantage of organizing health care workers is that those workers are not without financial resources, are motivated by ethical concerns, and exist in a seller's market for their services, so they don't really have to be afraid for their jobs. Health care workers can fund our organizing efforts if enough contribute and if we choose issues that inflame and focus their existing passion to put patients before profit. Because health care workers control the means of profit production, they can bring the market enterprise to its knees with select job actions that are designed to disrupt cash flow without impacting patient care. Want to get community control of a "nonprofit" hospital board that overpays its executive staff? The health care community can declare a boycott of one hospital in a market. Want to fix a useless, poorly designed electronic medical record that works to support billing but doesn't provide clinicians with the information they need? Have the majority of users in that hospital and clinic start handwriting their notes.

There are many opportunities for health care workers to revolt, redesign their own work, and begin to create a health care system place by place and institution by institution. Each victory will tilt the health care enterprise toward people and away from profit, and each victory will embolden this critical sector of the population, so that health care workers, who know health care best, can start doing the work their hearts are yearning to do, which is to build a health care system that serves all Americans, and that serves them well, so that we can be proud of this nation again because of what it does for its people as one nation, indivisible, after all.

When a hundred doctors or nurses appear in scrubs or white coats on the steps of a statehouse, people listen. When a million health care workers march on Washington, the nation listens. These are all opportunities to call attention to aspects of the wealth extraction system that are hardest to bear. Luxury suites in hospitals for board members and their friends, but overcrowded hallways staffed by overworked nurses for the rest of us. Rate hikes from insurance companies and unnecessary paperwork or computerized information that diverts the attention of nurses or doctors from their patients can and must be called out, but this is not just an opportunity to focus on the paperwork: we'll also use every opportunity to call out the profits and salaries of investors and executives, remembering that when one investor or executive has a dollar she or he didn't work for, one patient has a moment when they needed someone to hear them and there wasn't anyone there.

Once upon a time, primary care doctors went to the hospital every day and cared for their patients when they needed hospitalization. It was a better system than the system of hospitalists we have now. Every patient had someone they knew and trusted to take care of them when they were in the hospital, and that made the transition from hospital to home a smooth one—the person who took care of you in the hospital also took care of you at home, so you and your doctor both knew what had transpired in the hospital and what you would need at home afterward. The system was hard on doctors, though, because we had to be thinking about patients in the community and patients in the hospital at the same time. As hospital care involved more and more technology, it became harder and harder to keep up with the pace of that care. Insurance companies didn't help, because they failed to recognize the value of having one clinician taking care of people both at home and in the hospital, so they failed to develop a method to pay clinicians fairly for the time we spent in hospitals.

In that period, I worked in an academic hospital that no longer cared whether primary care doctors took care of their own patients in the hospital every day. A number of that hospital's doctors argued for a system, which then would have cost $1 million a year, to provide each patient with a physician assistant or nurse practitioner to do much of the mechanical work of patient care (writing orders and coordinating tests and results), so that a patient's primary care doctor could see the patient quickly and efficiently and still get to their office on time. The hospital decided that such a system was too expensive and never implemented it. Too expensive, at $1 million a year for almost all the patients in the hospital. What they didn't say but I learned later was that at the same time we were talking about this system, the hospital's CEO was earning $3 million a year. The hospital could have afforded it if they had paid their CEO less. The CEO would have made only $2 million a year, and patients would have had better service and seen their own doctor, someone they knew and hopefully trusted, every day.

The failure to implement the system I and others proposed meant that primary care doctors stopped coming to the hospital and turned over the care of their hospitalized patients to hospitalists who didn't know each patient very well and wouldn't care for these patients after they left the hospital. The emergence of the hospitalist system in health care created a new set of very serious problems for people who used the hospital—problems that occur after hospitalized patients are discharged, because their primary care doctors, who care for them in their homes and their communities, haven't been involved with their hospitalization, don't know what medications they are on or why, and can't give those patient's intelligent advice if they have more problems.

If I had known then what I know now, we would have organized the hospital's primary care doctors, appeared before the hospital board or organized a little demonstration at the main entrance, and fought until the hospital created a system that spent money on patients instead of funding the bank account of that hospital's CEO. And if we had stood up and created a little demonstration in front of the hospital, everyone in the community and in the state would have learned then about money in health care and would have learned that when one person has a dollar they didn't work for, some other person has a service they didn't get.

Health care workers also bring with them a powerful opportunity to mobilize the public in support of the Movement for Health Care in America. Health care workers see millions of people a day in one-on-one interactions in exam rooms, in hospital rooms, in laboratories, and in radiology suites. We are trusted by the people we take care of, because the public realizes that we put people before profit. It is now time to leverage that opportunity and earn back that trust by talking to the people we take care of in exam rooms. Health care is for people, not for profit. We don't need more reform of the insurance market. Insurance and markets are problems, not the solution. We need a health care system that cares for every American in every community. Let's take a moment. I'll tell you what a real health care system is, how it works, and why it would be better for everyone. Help us organize it.

There are lots of opportunities for little job actions, boycotts, and demonstrations by health care professionals and people in communities. Whenever a hospital eliminates a needed community service, there is an opportunity for people to organize and speak out. Whenever a hospital board gives its hospital CEO a million-dollar raise or a fat bonus, there is an opportunity for the community to boycott that hospital until the board is restructured and its members elected by the community it serves. Whenever a health insurance company raises its rates (again), there is an opportunity for health care workers to collaborate with small businesses and people who have to pay for their own insurance to organize, speak out, and take their business elsewhere—or organize their own little health care system that is not for profit but prioritizes primary care and prevention and is therefore likely to be much more affordable. Whenever an insurer or CMS imposes another new requirement, there is an opportunity for health care workers to mobilize patients affected and for clinicians and their patients to organize and speak out together. Whenever Medicare creates a new charge or a new complexity (again), there is an opportunity for health care work-ers to mobilize elderly people to speak out. Job actions and dem-onstrations are hard to pull off because the people who might participate are busy and don't want to be impolite. But with a little mutual support and a little knowledge and forethought, we can keep the public's attention on how the health care market has failed us, and as we do so continuously stress that we have a medical services market, not a health care system, but that together we can build a health care system for Americans, which is to say, for people and not for profit.

And, truth be told, we need to remind ourselves over and over that there is nothing more impolite than what is being done to the American people in the name of health care.

Market power works for those who create critical mass. Social power—the ability to change how we organize ourselves—works exactly the same way. United we stand. So let's unite, stand up together, build us a health care system, and reinvigorate our democracy.

Building Small Health Care Systems in Every Community

The health care reform efforts of 1993 and 2009-2010 were run by large national organizations that used orthodox processes to change the way the federal government deals with health care. Politics, it is said, is the art of the possible, and the result that was finally achieved in 2010 (which more or less got the reform that was designed in 1993 by a bipartisan group of senators) is likely all that is possible using the legislative processes of the federal government. And that wasn't good enough.

So perhaps we need to think about building the Movement for Health Care in America differently. Large national organizations failed us. So we'll start the Movement for Health Care in America by building small local associations, and then bring those small organizations into large coalitions. Let's look for a moment at other models of systems that bring services to all Americans. Public education, the police, fire protection, public water systems, public sanitation, and even the U.S. mail all started the same way. They started with local efforts—with communities designing solutions for themselves. Some communities built local schools. Others created police departments. Still others created different versions of fire protection. Each used a different way of organizing the services and created different ways of spreading the cost. Some worked by subscription initially—you got fire protection in some places only if you paid for it. Others designed fire protection for every household and paid for it out of tax dollars. The same approach was true of city water, and even roads. In some places city water was a private enterprise, and you got it only if you paid to hook up to it. In other places, the first good roads were built privately and you paid a toll to use them. Some communities did this better than other communities. Not all communities got involved. But eventually people recognized that public education, public water and sewage, roads, the police, and fire protection were public services, and most communities came on board, funded all these services centrally, and supplied them to every household. Eventually, state and federal regulation, and then state and federal (mostly federal) funding, made sure all the approaches were safe and effective. Then state and federal funding was used to tie local approaches together into a single system that offered very similar services to all Americans and to enable communities that hadn't yet developed those services for their citizens to do so.

Health care is no different. Health care—at least primary health care—is an essential service. Shame on us that it has taken us all so long to figure this out.

To create the Movement for Health Care in America, we can all start where we live.

I live in Scituate, Rhode Island, a little exurban town of ten thousand, about fifteen miles from the city, which for us is

Providence, Rhode Island. Twenty years ago, I started talking and listening and finding people who thought there was something we could do together. I gave them the numbers and then got out of the way while people worked together. We spend almost $100 million a year on health care for the people who live in Scituate. No one knew that. Almost all of that money leaves town. No one knew that either. People who live in Scituate have about seventy-five babies a year. Those babies are delivered by sixty different doctors. Their mothers travel hither and yon all over the state when they are pregnant. No one knew that either. But everyone in Scituate knows those facts now.

Fifteen years ago, Scituate became the first community in the U.S. to guarantee all its residents access to primary medical and dental care. We got a little foundation money to get that started, and now the very Republican town government contributes every year to make sure every person in Scituate has health care. We are one of the best-vaccinated places in the county. People get flu shots when they go to vote and when they walk around the streets doing their Christmas shopping in December. Our kids get sports physicals in the fall at the school. We just built a Neighborhood Health Station at the little shopping plaza in the middle of town, a primary care center that aims to care for everyone in town, like the primary care centers described in Chapter 5. It has primary care doctors and dentists and will eventually be open from 8:00 a.m. to 8:00 p.m. weekdays and from 9:00 a.m. to 5:00 p.m. on weekends. We still have challenges—our town financial meeting has dwindled to the point that only about a hundred people out of six thousand voters come every year.[1] There are three different volunteer

---

1   Except in 2107! When five hundred people showed up to fight for the reversal of a town council decision to remove three hundred thousand dollars from the school department budget. Oddly, that happened about six months after the Neighborhood Health Station opened. Completely coincidental, to be sure, but suggestively coincidental.

ambulance corps that waste time and money competing with one another to serve the community—so there is room for our cooperation and democracy to improve. But working together we have accomplished a lot over twenty years. Other communities can and will do the same. It will look a little different in each place. In some places it will be stronger and in others weaker, but that diversity is good for us all, because that is how we learn.

In 2013, I met James Diossa, the young mayor of Central Falls, Rhode Island, the poorest city in one of the poorest states in New England. Central Falls is an old industrial city, just a little more than one square mile in area, and one of the most densely populated places in the U.S. It has always been an immigrant destination—first Irish and then French Canadian and Syrian and Polish and Columbian and Central American—and is now 70 percent Spanish-speaking. Central Falls went bankrupt in 2011, after most of the mills left and took most of the jobs with them. It lost its community center and a good deal of its pride in the process, but it also lost a decades-old corrupt city administration that ran city government for its own benefit and ignored most of the people who live in the city.

In 2013, along with the mayor and Mario Bueno, who runs a great community advocacy organization called Progreso Latino, I attended a community meeting called by the Rhode Island Department of Health to listen to what people were thinking and feeling about health and health care in Central Falls. We heard people saying that they wanted better access to primary care—more doctors who were open more hours—and better opportunities to be physically active, opportunities that had vanished when the bankrupt city lost its community center. As we walked out together, the mayor, Mario, and I wondered out loud how we could help, how we could make things a little better. So we did what people in government sometimes do when we don't know the answer. We called a meeting and got lots of people who live or work in Central Falls and who think about health and health care around a table.

And then wild things began to happen. People started working together.

First some of us figured out how to open a little clinic in the high school to make sure kids got vaccinations and contraception, because Central Falls had the highest rate of adolescent pregnancy in the state (four times the state average!). Then the local community health center took over a hospital-owned urgent care center that was located across a parking lot and that was competing with it for patients. Now the community health center and the urgent care center are run collaboratively as part of a single clinic enterprise. The urgent care center sees people who aren't patients of the community health center when they are sick, and the community health center follows up on patients that the urgent care center saw just once. Then the YMCA began running buses into Central Falls three times a week, so everyone in Central Falls has access to a place to exercise in the winter and to a swimming pool in the summer. A local foundation and AmeriCorps funded four community health workers to knock on doors and reach out to people who are ill but don't know how to find a doctor. The local housing authority gave those community health workers a place to work. That housing authority helps house people who are homeless or housing-insecure, whom it hears about from the community health workers. The health center sees patients from the housing authority, many of whom are frail and elderly. A large group called the Central Falls Neighborhood Health Center Multidisciplinary Team now gets together once a week on Friday to figure out how to care for people in Central Falls who are sick and in trouble. This team includes everyone in Central Falls who is concerned with the health and welfare of people the town—doctors and nurses, community health workers, mental and behavioral health agencies, insurance company medical directors, recovery specialists, physical therapists, home health nurses, legal aid lawyers, EMTs, and even the Community Service Unit of the Central Falls Police. We just broke ground on a $15 million building to house the new Central Falls Neighborhood Health Station, which will employ a hundred or more residents and will spark a new identity for the city, new hope and new energy, as we rebuild the economy of Central Falls by empowering the people to take care of one another.

As a result of this work, which began in the last year, ambulance runs have dropped 7 to 15 percent, and the number of high school girls getting pregnant dropped by 25 percent, preventing a cycle of poverty for fifteen families. And that's just the start. We aim to reduce ambulance runs by 50 percent, adolescent pregnancy by 80 percent, drug overdose death by 50 percent, and total health care cost for people living in Central Falls by 30 percent. And we're succeeding.

And we will succeed. That's what people can do when they work together. We *can* build health care systems from the ground up.

There are as many opportunities for people to collaborate in the U.S. as there are communities of ten to twenty thousand people. All across America, there are community health centers and small private primary care practices that function in the public interest, although those private practices receive no direct public funding to pay for their public health efforts. Each community health center and primary care practice builds a little health care system around itself. They build a list of specialists they trust, who will see their patients, the insured and the uninsured. They figure out how to get medicine for people who can't afford it. They figure out how to get mental health, substance use disorder, and alcohol use disorder treatment for people who need it. They work to find home health services for people who are homebound, even though home health has become a messy for-profit industry. They figure out how to get medical equipment like nebulizers, oxygen, hospital beds, walkers, and canes for people who need them. They learn to work with emergency medical services, so they can get ambulances for people when necessary. They often figure out how to arrange transportation for people too old, poor, or frail to arrange their own. They work out arrangements with nursing homes and hospitals, so they can move people in and out of those places, making sure people get the medicines and treatments they need and ensuring that primary care clinicians actually know what is going on with the patients they care for.

These small, de facto health care systems often involve fifty or a hundred health care workers of various stripes when they are all counted and represent substantial economic activity, as much as 25 percent of the economic activity of rural areas, and the expenditure of many millions of dollars.

The Movement for Health Care in America has the opportunity to begin organizing de facto systems into real systems, each with a mission, vision, values, and goals, each caring for ten thousand people in a community, and each convening weekly to make sure everyone is up to date on the people in the community whose care the clinicians and the other health workers share. These multidisciplinary teams will improve patient care. They will also allow health care workers from different professions to know and trust one another and prepare them to work together so that every person in each community is cared for. Once multidisciplinary teams are assembled, their combined data systems will allow them to identify who has been left out and needs to be reached. Once clinicians are working together, they create efficiencies that free up time to include those people who aren't connected or have excluded themselves. And once these multidisciplinary teams begin to trust one another, they can create messaging for all to use when they talk to patients.

People in many communities will perk up their ears, organize around the small health care systems, and open the political space we need to get the small health care systems funded in a way that is for people and not for profit, if all the health care workers say, over and over again: "We can build a health care system for the U.S. that includes everyone, actually improves our health, and saves us a trillion dollars a year. We are building a health care system here in our community. Learn about it. Here's how you can help." Then, as people get involved, they will be able to pressure their representatives in Congress and the state legislatures, who together can to write coherent enabling legislation to build a health care system that serves all Americans. This combination of local action, building local infrastructure first, and then building a national movement is how we got civil rights, how we ended the war in Vietnam, how we got universal public education, safe water and sewage treatment, and even how we created an infrastructure for public safety. Everyone is tired of hearing politicians and pundits who don't know anything about health care run their mouths. Now it is time for health care workers in their own communities to collaborate with their patients and their friends and lead this change.

Small health care systems are already starting to spring up around the nation. They have different forms and different names. You can see them in New Orleans and San Francisco and Maine, in Camden, New Jersey, and in the region around Albany, New York. They're in Southeast Alaska and in San Antonio, Texas, in Central Falls, Rhode Island, and in the Bronx and Manhattan and north along the Hudson River. They are being built by community health centers, by groups of primary care doctors, by cities and towns with visionary mayors and city councils, and by many others. The small health care systems that already exist were not built by pundits, think tanks, foundations, health policy experts (whose expertise is in admiring the problem), hospitals, health insurance companies, medical schools, or schools of public health, despite those organizations sucking down most of the money we spend on health.

In red states, the Movement for Health Care in America is likely to start in rural areas, which often already have little health care systems that function pretty much as I've described. In small towns, the population often only supports one primary care group for every ten thousand people, one home health agency, one emergency medical service, and one little hospital where there is physician therapy, home health, and mental and behavioral health. In those places, people are used to taking care of one another, regardless of what kind of insurance they have or don't have and regardless of the immigration status of people who are sick. In those rural areas, where costs tend to be lower, all it takes is a little education about what the health care profiteers are costing the community before people understand and can think about keeping more of that wasted (or stolen) money for themselves. In those places, communities can develop rural co-ops to help everyone in a community create and fund health savings accounts—a very Republican idea with great public health potential—as a vehicle to fund the kind of prevention that all communities need. HSAs can be used to pay for primary care by the month, a process that, when done intelligently and fairly, allows each primary care center to care for everyone in the community and remain financially sound.

Blue states may well just go ahead and build single-payer systems for primary care. They can create funds consolidators—sometimes called primary care trusts—to purchase expanded primary care services from community health centers and larger private practices.[2] Paying for those services by the month and

---

2   "Primary care trust" is also a term used in the UK to describe local and regional fund holders for all health care services. The British primary care trusts are closer to our health maintenance organizations. I'm using the term "primary care trust" here to describe state organizations that buy

paying for them fairly will give states the leverage they need to create a more robust and standardized approach to primary care than we have now, and they can use the flow of funds through these purchase programs to seed the building of one clinical entity for every ten thousand people and to help pay for the training of more primary care clinicians.

In both red states and blue states it will take that same process of exposing, educating, revolting, and collaborating to build small and then larger health care systems. This process will require true movement building, with people in each community learning from one another and building on the experiences of different communities and states. Red states and blue states may approach the process differently, but the movement will move forward over many years if the people collaborating keep their eyes on the prize.

Organizing a National Movement

We'll need to organize ourselves into a national coordinating council if we are going to spread this message.

First, we'll need to convene the national organizations whose members have an interest in containing health care costs, making sure we have a healthy workforce, and improving the public's health. The National League of Cities and Towns, the National Small Business Association, the National Association of Community Health Centers, National Nurses United and the National Federation of Nurses, SEIU and UNITE HERE, the American Association of Family Physicians, the American Academy of Pediatricians, the American College of Physicians, the American Academy of Physician Assistants, and the American

---

primary care for a state's entire population, using tax dollars for Medicaid patients and Medicare patients and scooping the primary care budget out of each person's health insurance plan, thereby becoming the payer for the health insurance process. Primary care trust-enabling legislation was introduced in the Vermont and Rhode Island legislatures in 2018.

Association of Nurse Practitioners all should have an interest in this movement, but they haven't, in general, been change agents. Our challenge is to bring these and other organizations together and help them understand what a health care system looks like and how a health care system for the U.S. can save money while it improves the public's health and strengthens communities. Once we've built a national coordinating council, we'll have to agree on the message and the messaging, so we will enlist their membership in every city and town in the U.S. to say over and over: "We can build a health care system for the U.S. that includes everyone, actually improves our health, and saves us a trillion dollars a year. We are building a health care system in our communities. Learn about it. Here's how you can help."

In a certain way, presidential campaigns, as painful as they were to watch in 2016, provide an excellent example of how to motivate a large number of people to achieve a specific result. Presidential campaigns use a single unifying image—the candidate—to create focus. Then they employ both traditional marketing—social media and television and radio commercials—and hundreds of surrogates in every neighborhood and community to both inflame the imagination and facilitate action on the ground to get people to the polls. We'll need to build that kind of campaign around a single unifying image, which is a health care system that cares for all Americans. Then we'll need a stump speech and a few dedicated whistle-stompers traveling the country, exposing, educating, inciting, and imagining, so that our health care worker organizing and the work of local communities building small health care systems for themselves feed a central, national conversation about how to end the medical services marketplace and finally build a health care system.

The process of understanding how health care has been used to transfer public assets to private pocketbooks, and then turning that understanding into action as communities start to create small health care systems for themselves, has been called *critical consciousness* and helps us create a way to measure our progress. We'll be able to say the Movement for Health Care in America is successful when we can count communities that have built small health care systems and count the number of people who those small health systems serve. We'll be able to enlist more people and more communities when we can show how the measured public health (infant mortality, life expectancy, and preventable years of life lost) is improving and the cost of health care dropping wherever communities have built small health care systems for themselves. When we show how there is more social trust in those places, more participation in book clubs and softball leagues and parent-teacher associations, when we can prove that income inequality drops and health disparities on the basis of race disappear, and when voter participation goes up, more communities will jump on board, and it will be easier to enlist more states and Congress to write the legislation needed to spread this approach to every neighborhood, city, and town in the U.S.

The health care profiteers, the haters, and the doubters will be present all along the way, shouting about choice and death panels and socialized medicine and other fictions that can be used to drive people to buy what they don't need and what can hurt them. And those profiteers, haters, and doubters have billions of dollars to spend to distract people, in the hope they can still profit at public expense.

That's why telling the story of each community and each small health system is so important. Because every time a hater or a doubter makes up a lie about how the market is the only way to sell health and health care, they are trying to convince Americans that democracy doesn't matter, even though none of us—no neighborhood, community, patient, health professional, or even any of the haters or doubters—none of all the people who will benefit from a health care system will have much of a life if the haters and doubters convince the rest of us to take democracy apart.

And while we are telling the story of each small health system and of the multiclinics and hospitals we assemble to make a health care system, we also need to tell ourselves the story of our democracy and celebrate that democracy, which will allow this health care revolt and make health care happen in America again. If we succeed, it is because we used our democracy, which is still our greatest achievement. Democracy makes us strong, able, and healthy, and democracy matters way more than one drug or treatment or hospital ever can.

It will take ten or twenty years to turn America's attention to what health is, and another ten or twenty years to build a health care system out of our chaotic marketplace. Along the way, we'll have to deal with government waste and inefficiency, the distorted power of public employee unions, the various types of health professionals who will battle with one another for turf, the usual swarm of lobbyists who will try to subvert the legislative and regulatory process in the service of private profit, the egos and lusts and workplace dramas that come to bear whenever Americans have to work together, and a host of haters who think they believe that America was made great by individual initiative instead of collective action (but really believe only in selfishness and greed).

But *if* we keep our eyes on the prize, *if* we can remember that democracy is the process we use to keep our lusts and egos from destroying civil society, *if* we can remember that the health of individuals is a necessary condition of democracy, *if* we can help others understand that the public's health is the way we measure democracy's success, and *if* we can convince others that a health care system exists to strengthen individuals so they can participate in the democratic process and *not* to create private profit, *if* we can remember all those ideas, goals, and aspirations, then we will be able to build a health care system that strengthens democracy as it attends to the needs of individuals and improves public health.

That's a lot of big *ifs* and a long and winding road. But though success will be difficult to achieve, it is also impossible for us to fail. It is hard to imagine health care much worse than what we have today, where the market for medical services and the market generally is being used to sell what is harmful, and the profits those markets generate are being used to undermine the democratic process. By working together to make a health care system, we'll create healthy communities and resuscitate democracy, all at the same time. Is all this likely? Of course it isn't. But was human life likely? Was democracy likely? All of this is just a dream. We are all dreamers, but here we are. The Movement for Health Care in America is impossible—unless we build it.

But we can dream together. And learn to act together. And perhaps make even this dream come true.

That's what a health care system is for and *that's* what democracy looks like.

CHAPTER EIGHT

Why Clinicians Must Revolt

THE NEED FOR CLINICIAN REVOLT SPRINGS FROM OUR OWN EXPERIENCE OF EX-
ploitation and dehumanization. Once upon a time, the special
intimacy between clinicians and patients was the secret sauce
of healing, the connection we leveraged to help people cope and
change and grow. That intimacy was the deeply human moment
that nourished us through the long nights on call, that helped us
recover from the raw terror that we feel at the moment a baby is
born, knowing the baby may or may not breathe and the mother
may or may not bleed out—until a crying newborn is placed, still
wet, on its mother's chest to suckle. That intimacy sustained
us through the bottomless moments when a patient's life was
slipping away, as the body failed but the love of their families
and our quiet confidence made the transition from life to death
a safe one and their loss survivable.

That intimacy is for patients, but it is also for us. It is what
brought us to health care in the first place. It's why we are
nurses, doctors, nurse practitioners, and physician assistants,
not lawyers, venture capitalists, and accountants. It is exactly
that intimacy that the market has stolen from us by turning us
into machines to crank out patient encounters. That intimacy
once gave our professional lives meaning.

Once we worked only for the patients and communities
we cared for. Now we work for hospitals or hospital systems,
for large practices, large community health centers, or large
HMOs, and those organizations have contracts with government,

with insurers, with other health systems. Each of those other entities has its own contracts with pharmaceutical companies and device manufacturers and medical equipment companies and substance use treatment facilities and mental health organizations, with layers upon layers of organizations that purport to organize and manage care, so we each end up with virtual contracts with thousands of businesses and organizations that are not the patient and community we thought we signed up to care for. The uncomfortable truth is that we have all been bought off. The world is changing. It costs lots of money to send kids to college. You need to put money into a 401(k) if you ever want to retire. The media teaches that you ought to have a nice car and live in a comfortable house in a safe community. We each learned how to find a safe job that paid a certain amount of money and brought with it certain benefits, and even how to negotiate for a better salary, less call, better benefits, and some dedicated time for research, writing, and teaching. With that job and those deals came rules and regulations that you have to swallow if you want to keep the job. A certain number of patients per hour. You have to fill out this form and that form, even when the forms are confusing and meaningless. You have to sit at the computer and check off the boxes, instead of sitting on the edge of the patient's bed and listening to the person. You go home at night and live in a neighborhood with big houses and other people who go home at night to live in a neighborhood with big houses, none of which was what you intended to do when you went to health professional school in the first place.

Any of us could have revolted at any point along the way. We could have refused to take a couple of crappy insurance plans and not had to swallow some of the forms and the preauthorizations or the limited formularies and networks. We could have, but we didn't want to lose patients who got switched to that insurance, and one part of us always wanted to be sure we had more new patients so we could cover the overhead and maintain our incomes, even if we had to compromise to do that. We could have revolted when CMS designed some new form or idiotic new procedure that made no sense and stopped taking Medicare until Congress fixed it. We could have refused to use the clunky inelegant and disconnected electronic medical record systems that have been forced on us over the last twenty years—systems that cost a zillion dollars, don't improve patient care, and increase our workload to the point that many of us go home after a long day of work and work late into the night. We could have revolted against these electronic medical record systems that create profit for the companies that make them but haven't improved patient care one iota.

We could have organized, gone on strike, refused to comply with the zillions of bureaucracies invented by the green-visor guys who didn't know anything about the special loneliness of the sick. If we had revolted every step of the way, perhaps we would have slowed or stopped the transition to a market that is for profit. But we failed to act up, because, intentionally or not, we became for-profit ourselves.

Now we have to look at what our complicity has wrought. We have a market, not a health care system. Life expectancies for Americans are shrinking, not improving. Democracy itself is under attack, an attack fueled in part by money generated by the health care profiteers while we remained silent.

We now have a choice. We can either stand up and fight for our patients, their families, and our communities, or we can accept this new reality, as automatons in a market devoted to profit, as statues without hearts.

Clinicians have information that communities don't have. We know about health outcomes, and we know about costs. We experience every day what most people experience only once every few years or once in a lifetime: the costs and chaos that a disorganized marketplace produces for individuals who are sick.

Everyone now knows that if you have life-threatening allergies, for example, it is hard to spend $700 on an EpiPen that cost $40 ten years ago, and everyone is shocked, shocked that the price went up so much. But your doctor or your nurse practitioner or your physician assistant—that person sees someone struggle to pay for their EpiPen many times a week and has seen the cost of many generic drugs and prescription drugs shoot up over the last few years. The costs and chaos of the marketplace are always in clinicians' faces, and the examples of what has gone wrong are omnipresent for those of us who practice medicine. Those of us who see what's wrong have the responsibility to name the problem and lead the change. The defining principal of professionalism, non-self-interested advocacy, the requirement that we put the needs of our patients before our own needs, is the principle that requires clinicians to act, speak up, speak out, and revolt because of how intensely the medical services marketplace is failing the people we take care of.

Nurses have been *much* better at organizing than doctors. Nurses' unions have fought back against the speedups, crazy shifts, and work rules that endanger patient care, and by fighting back nurses' unions have made hospitals safer and more humane places. But no health profession can be effective alone. For a revolt to be effective, we all have to revolt together. An injury to one is an injury to all. *That's* what democracy looks like.

People listen to health professionals. That's the dynamic of our relationships. People tell us what they are worried about, and then they listen to us, hoping we will tell them what to do. People understand that we have expert knowledge that they might benefit from. And people have been waiting for two generations for us to tell them how to make a health care system.

We can and must revolt to defend our own lives and the relationships we hold dear. Revolt is now the only way we can honor our professional obligations. For-profit medicine is the disease, and a health care system that is focused on democracy is the treatment. We are health professionals, and patients listen to what we have to say about health and health care. Our job is to recognize the disease and to recommend treatment. Our revolt is part of that treatment, because only that revolt will help everyone understand how diseased we have become.

Money has been a taboo subject among health care profession-als, and health care workers have been afraid to talk about our own incomes, out of fear the public will think what we make is excessive—which it is. But until we come clean and hold our-selves accountable to the same standards we want to apply to others, no one will take us seriously. We'll have to talk about what we are making and be ready to give up some of that if we are going to be able to fix this mess. We will need to donate a part of what we make to the Movement for Health Care in America if that movement is going to succeed—and we'll end up getting paid less on the other end. To those who believe that the market is the solution for all things, paying up front for a process that will lead to our earning less will seem ludicrous.

But we all know that what we have is unsustainable. Isn't it better to give up $10,000 or $15,000 a year (for most of us, but much more for high-earning specialists and administrators) and build a health care system that serves every American and live in a place where we have justice and peace instead of in a nation that is bursting apart at the seams, as it is sucked into an downward spiral of unending partisan conflict?

What should our revolt look like?

First, we have to unionize. Nurses unionized long ago and the unions protected the professionalism of their members, making hospitals better and safer places. We need to think about and build a new kind of union, though, a union of all health professionals, not one that lets us be Balkanized by job title or professional training. Any health professional who is a salaried employee—now about 80 percent of clinicians—needs to join a union tomorrow, so that we have a voice. That voice needs to focus on preserving the intimacy of the relationship between health professionals and the patients we serve and not on increasing our incomes. Our unions need to call out the salaries and the profits of the health care profiteers, and we need to focus first on linkage—on linking the salaries of our lowest-paid colleagues with the salaries of executives, so that all our colleagues make a living wage.

Then we need to strike. But we must never stop patient care. Our strikes must focus on the stupid work that only enriches others. We can and must refuse to do the preauthorizations and preapprovals and to sign forms that don't matter. When one of us refuses, they can fire that one person. But they can't fire a million of us. They need us much more than we need them. We need to refuse, together, to use the electronic medical records until they change the software so that those computers free us to look at and listen to patients instead of looking at and listening to computer screens. Until they build us computerized records that support our work.

And we need to march. We need a million health professionals marching on Washington and demanding changes in the laws that allow pharmaceutical companies to gouge patients who are ill and their insurance companies, using publicly granted patents and licenses to create ungodly profits. We need to organize in our examining rooms, telling patients about how these corporate raiders exploit the legislative and regulatory process to make communities poorer and the rich richer, and then we can and must invite patients to join us when we march. This is a still a democracy. If the laws that govern us are being used against us, then we can and must change those laws and the lawmakers, until we get laws that protect patients and communities. Think we need to give the government the ability to negotiate prices with pharmaceutical companies? Think we need a public health insurance option? Worried about lobbyists? Put a hundred thousand people in front of every state capitol and a million people on the Capitol Mall and see how long it takes for those lobbyists to run and hide.

If we revolt, we will spark the development of a health care system built to strengthen a robust democracy. If we can bring our patients and our communities into our revolt, we'll put meaning back into democracy itself.

CHAPTER NINE
Health Care and Democracy

HEALTH CARE AND DEMOCRACY. DANCER AND DANCE. IT IS HARD TO KNOW which got out of whack first or what did what to whom. Health care became a for-profit business. Democracy was co-opted by the rich and powerful to serve themselves. We the people got distracted by stuff—by material goods and technology. We took our eyes off the road and our hands off the steering wheel.

History is littered with experiments in democracy and equality, with short periods of light during which people stand up for themselves and make a government of, by, and for the people. Human history is the story of the struggle to move from periods of relative darkness, when self-interest rules, to periods of relative light, when we see and value one another and when our politics, art, and culture congeal around the opportunity to be together and build together as one people.

If politics is the art of the possible, then the imagination is the home of our transformation from serving ourselves to working toward what is achievable together.

Some will say that nothing in this book is achievable. Others will say that these arguments are assumptions built on assumptions.

Dr. Don Berwick, who founded the Institute for Health Care Improvement, often says that each system was created to produce the results it produces. Democracy is a system designed to produce equality, justice, liberty, and happiness. Health care exists to allow individuals to experience that liberty and happiness, to fight for equality and justice, and to strengthen democracy in the process.

If our democracy is off the tracks and our health care has become about profit for the few instead of justice for the many, then it is time to revolt, make health care for people, not for profit, and bring life back into our democracy, while we still have enough freedom left to fight for what matters as free people.

For more than a millennium, democracy itself appeared unachievable, but then human beings acted and built it.

A health care revolt is unlikely, unless we act, act together, and act together soon.

Or, in the words of another time: yes we can.

Bibliography

Abramson, John. *Overdosed America: The Broken Promise of American Medicine*. New York: Harper Collins, 2004.

Alinsky, Saul. *Rules for Radicals: A Pragmatic Primer for Realistic Radicals*. New York: Vintage Books, 1971.

Angell, Marcia. *The Truth about the Drug Companies: How They Deceive Us and What to Do about It*. New York: Random House, 2004.

Beatley, Timothy, and Kristy Manning. *The Ecology of Place: Planning for Environment, Economy, and Community*. Washington, DC: Island Press, 1997.

Berkman Lisa F., and Ichiro Kawachi, eds. *Social Epidemiology*. Oxford: Oxford University Press, 2000.

Brill, Steven. *America's Bitter Pill: Money, Politics, Backroom Deals, and the Fight to Fix Our Broken Health Care System*. New York: Random House, 2015.

Brownlee, Shannon. *Overtreated: Why Too Much Medicine Is Making Us Sicker and Poorer*. New York: Bloomsbury, 2007.

Callahan, Daniel. *What Price Better Health? Hazards of the Research Imperative*. Berkeley: University of California Press, 2003.

Cardello, Hank, with Doug Garr. *Stuffed: An Insider's Look at Who's (Really) Making America Fat and How the Food Industry Can Fix It*. New York: Ecco, 2009.

Cutler, David. *Your Money or Your Life: Strong Medicine for America's Health Care System*. Oxford: Oxford University Press, 2004.

Daniels, Norman. *Just Health Care*. Cambridge: Cambridge University Press, 1985.

Daniels, Norman, Bruce Kennedy, and Ichiro Kawachi. *Is Inequality Bad for Our Health?* Boston: Beacon Press, 2000.

Davis, Karen, and Cathy Schoen. *Health and the War on Poverty: A Ten-Year Appraisal*. Washington, DC: Brookings Institution, 1978.

Dubos, René. *Mirage of Health: Utopias, Progress and Biological Change*. New Brunswick, NJ: Rutgers University Press, 1959.

Fine, Michael, and James W. Peters. *The Nature of Health: How America Lost, and Can Regain, a Basic Human Value.* Oxford: Radcliffe Publishing, 2007.

Fitzpatrick, Kevin, and Mark LaGory. *Unhealthy Places: The Ecology of Risk in the Urban Landscape.* New York: Routledge, 2000.

Freire, Paulo. *Pedagogy of the Oppressed.* New York: Continuum, 1970.

Freymann, John Gordon. *The American Health Care System: Its Genesis and Trajectory.* Malabar, FL: Krieger Publishing, 1974.

Fuchs, Victor R. *Who Shall Live? Health, Economics, and Social Choice.* New York: Basic Books, 1974.

Herzlinger, Regina. *Who Killed Health Care? America's $2 Trillion Medical Problem—and the Consumer-Driven Cure.* New York: McGraw Hill, 2007.

Institute of Medicine. *Primary Care: America's Health in a New Era.* Edited by Molla S. Donaldson et al. Washington, DC: National Academies Press, 1996.

Institute of Medicine. *Unequal Treatment: Confronting Racial and Ethnic Disparities in Healthcare.* Edited by Brian D. Smedley, Adrienne Y. Stith, and Alan R. Nelson. Washington, DC: National Academies Press, 2006.

Katcher, Avrum L. *A Time to Remember.* Flemington, NJ: Hunterdon Medical Center Foundation, 2003.

Kawachi, Ichiro, and Lisa F. Berkman. *Neighborhoods and Health.* Oxford: Oxford University Press, 2003.

Kawachi, Ichiro, and Bruce P. Kennedy. *The Health of Nations: Why Inequality Is Harmful to Your Health.* New York: New Press, 2002.

Kearns, Robert A., and Wilbert M. Gesler. *Putting Health into Place: Landscape, Identity and Well-Being.* Syracuse: Syracuse University Press, 1998.

Kleinke, J.D. *Oxymorons: The Myth of a U.S. Health Care System.* San Francisco: Jossey-Bass, 2001.

Kretzmann, John P., and John L. McKnight. *Building Communities from the Inside Out: A Path Toward Finding and Mobilizing a Community's Assets.* Chicago: ACTA Publications, 1993.

Marmot, Michael. *The Status Syndrome: How Social Standing Affects Our Health and Longevity.* New York: Henry Holt, 2004.

Marmot, Michael, and Richard Wilkinson, eds. *Social Determinants of Health.* Oxford: Oxford University Press, 1999.

McKeown, Thomas. *The Role of Medicine: Dream, Mirage, or Nemesis?.* Princeton, NJ: Princeton University Press, 1979.

McKnight, John. *The Careless Society: Community and Its Counterfeits.* New York: Basic Books, 1995.

Minkler, Meredith, ed. *Community Organizing and Community Building for Health*. New Brunswick, NJ: Rutgers University Press, 1997.

Peterson, M.A. "Kenneth Arrow and the Changing Economics of Health Care." *Journal of Health Politics, Policy and Law* 26, no. 5 (October 2001): 823-28.

Putnam, Robert D. *Bowling Alone: The Collapse and Revival of American Community*. New York: Simon & Schuster, 2000.

Reid, T.R. *The Healing of America: A Global Quest for Better, Cheaper, and Fairer Health Care*. New York: Penguin Books, 2009.

Rosenthal, Elisabeth. *An American Sickness: How Healthcare Became Big Business and How You Can Take It Back*. New York: Penguin Books, 2017.

Rothman, David J., ed. *Combating Conflict of Interest: A Primer for Countering Industry Marketing*. New York: Institute on Medicine as a Profession, 2012.

Rothman, David J. *Strangers at the Bedside: A History of How Law and Bioethics Transformed Medical Decision Making*. New York: Basic Books, 1991.

Shi, Leiyu, and Douglas A. Singh. *Delivering Health Care in America: A Systems Approach*. Gaithersburg, MD: Aspen Publishers, 2001.

Shi, Leiyu, and Gregory D. Stevens. *Vulnerable Populations in the United States*. San Francisco: Jossey-Bass, 2005.

Starfield, Barbara. *Primary Care: Balancing Health Needs, Services, and Technology*. New York: Oxford University Press, 1998.

Starr, Paul. *The Social Transformation of American Medicine*. New York: Basic Books, 1982.

Stevens, Rosemary. *American Medicine and the Public Interest: A History of Specialization*. Berkeley: University of California Press, 1971.

Stevens, Rosemary. *In Sickness and in Health: American Hospitals in the Twentieth Century*. New York: Basic Books, 1989.

Stiglitz, Joseph E. *The Great Divide: Unequal Societies and What We Can Do about Them*. New York: WW Norton, 2015.

Ward, Thomas J., Jr. *Out in the Rural: A Mississippi Health Center and Its War on Poverty*. New York: Oxford University Press, 2017.

Wilkinson, Richard G. *Unhealthy Societies*. London: Routledge, 1996.

Wolf, Stewart, and John G. Bruhn. *The Power of Clan: The Influence of Human Relationships on Heart Disease*. New Brunswick, NJ: Transaction Publishers, 1993.

About the Author

Michael Fine, MD, is chief health strategist for the City of Central Falls, Rhode Island, and senior population health and clinical services officer at Blackstone Valley Health Care, Inc. Fine guides a partnership between the City and Blackstone that created the Central Falls Neighborhood Health Station, the first attempt in the U.S. to build a population-based primary care and public health collaboration that serves the entire population of a particular locale. Dr. Fine served in the cabinet of Governor Lincoln Chafee as Director of the Rhode Island Department of Health (HEALTH) from February 2011 until March 2015, where he was responsible for a broad range of public health programs and services, oversaw 450 public health professionals, and managed a budget of $110 million a year.

Dr. Fine's career as both a family physician and manager in the field of health care has been devoted to health care reform, with a particular focus on underserved populations. Before his confirmation as director of health, Dr. Fine was the medical program director at the Rhode Island Department of Corrections, overseeing a health care unit servicing nearly twenty thousand people a year, with a staff of over eighty-five physicians, psychiatrists, mental health workers, nurses, and other health professionals. He was a founder and managing director of HealthAccessRI, the nation's first statewide organization making prepaid, reduced fee-for-service primary care available to people without employer-provided health insurance.

Dr. Fine practiced for sixteen years in urban Pawtucket, Rhode Island, and rural Scituate, Rhode Island. He is the former physician operating officer of Hillside Avenue Family and Community Medicine, the largest family practice in Rhode Island, and the former physician-in-chief of the Rhode Island and Miriam

Hospitals' Departments of Family and Community Medicine. He was co-chair of the Allied Advocacy Group for Integrated Primary Care. He convened and facilitated the Primary Care Leadership Council, a statewide organization that represented 75 percent of Rhode Island's primary care physicians and practices. He currently serves on the boards of Crossroads Rhode Island, the state's largest service organization for the homeless, the Lown Institute, the George Wiley Center, and RICARES.

Dr. Fine founded the Scituate Health Alliance, a community-based, population-focused nonprofit organization, which made Scituate the first community in the United States to provide primary medical and dental care to all town residents. Dr. Fine is a past president of the Rhode Island Academy of Family Physicians and was an Open Society Institute / George Soros Fellow in Medicine as a Profession from 2000 to 2002. He has served on a number of legislative committees for the Rhode Island General Assembly, has chaired the Primary Care Advisory Committee for the Rhode Island Department of Health, and sat on both the Urban Family Medicine Task Force of the American Academy of Family Physicians and the National Advisory Council to the National Health Services Corps.

Dr. Fine is the coauthor, with James W. Peters, of *The Nature of Health* (Oxford: Radcliffe, 2007), a study of health care services, human rights, society, technology, and industry. Dr. Fine is also the author of *The Zero Calorie Diet* (North Springfield, VT: Red House Press, 2010), a look at the culture of excess through the lens of fasting.

Dr. Fine's career prior to and just after becoming a physician shaped his view of community health care. His early professional experience included jobs as a printer, a metalworker, a New York City taxi driver, and a VISTA volunteer and community health organizer in the South Bronx. As a National Health Services Corps Scholar in the mid-1980s, Fine worked for three years in rural Tennessee, in the fifth-poorest county in America. In that community, with an illiteracy rate of 60 percent, he experienced the inextricable links between education and health, income and health, and health care and local economic development.

Dr. Fine lives in Scituate, Rhode Island, with his wife Carol Levitt, also a family physician.

Index

"Passim" (literally "scattered") indicates intermittent discussion of a topic over a cluster of pages.

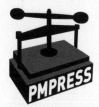

About PM Press

politics • culture • art • fiction • music • film

PM Press was founded at the end of 2007 by a small collection of folks with decades of publishing, media, and organizing experience. PM Press co-conspirators have published and distributed hundreds of books, pamphlets, CDs, and DVDs. Members of PM have founded enduring book fairs, spearheaded victorious tenant organizing campaigns, and worked closely with bookstores, academic conferences, and even rock bands to deliver political and challenging ideas to all walks of life. We're old enough to know what we're doing and young enough to know what's at stake.

We create radical and stimulating fiction and nonfiction books, pamphlets, T-shirts, visual and audio materials to educate, entertain, and inspire. We aim to distribute these through every available channel with every available technology, whether that means you are seeing anarchist classics at our bookfair stalls; reading our latest vegan cookbook at the café; downloading geeky fiction e-books; or digging new music and timely videos from our website.

Contact us for direct ordering and questions about all PM Press releases, as well as manuscript submissions, review copy requests, foreign rights sales, author interviews, to book an author for an event, and to have PM Press attend your bookfair:

PM Press
PO Box 23912
Oakland, CA 94623
510-658-3906 • info@pmpress.org

PM Press in Europe
europe@pmpress.org
www.pmpress.org.uk

Buy books and stay on top of what we are doing at:

www.pmpress.org

1-19

FOPM

MONTHLY SUBSCRIPTION PROGRAM

These are indisputably momentous times—the financial system is melting down globally and the Empire is stumbling. Now more than ever there is a vital need for radical ideas.

In the ten years since its founding—and on a mere shoestring—PM Press has risen to the formidable challenge of publishing and distributing knowledge and entertainment for the struggles ahead. With over 450 releases to date, we have published an impressive and stimulating array of literature, art, music, politics, and culture. Using every available medium, we've succeeded in connecting those hungry for ideas and information to those putting them into practice.

Friends of PM allows you to directly help impact, amplify, and revitalize the discourse and actions of radical writers, filmmakers, and artists. It provides us with a stable foundation from which we can build upon our early successes and provides a much-needed subsidy for the materials that can't necessarily pay their own way. You can help make that happen—and receive every new title automatically delivered to your door once a month—by joining as a Friend of PM Press. And, we'll throw in a free T-Shirt when you sign up.

Here are your options:
- $30 a month: Get all books and pamphlets plus 50% discount on all webstore purchases
- $40 a month: Get all PM Press releases (including CDs and DVDs) plus 50% discount on all webstore purchases
- $100 a month: Superstar—Everything plus PM merchandise, free downloads, and 50% discount on all webstore purchases

For those who can't afford $30 or more a month, we have **Sustainer Rates** at $15, $10 and $5. Sustainers get a free PM Press T-shirt and a 50% discount on all purchases from our website.

Your Visa or Mastercard will be billed once a month, until you tell us to stop. Or until our efforts succeed in bringing the revolution around. Or the financial meltdown of Capital makes plastic redundant. Whichever comes first.